First Aid

An Illustrated
Teach Yourself book

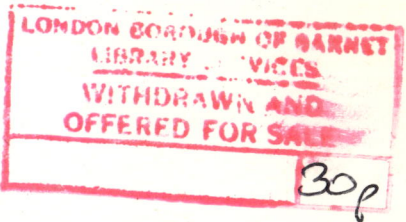

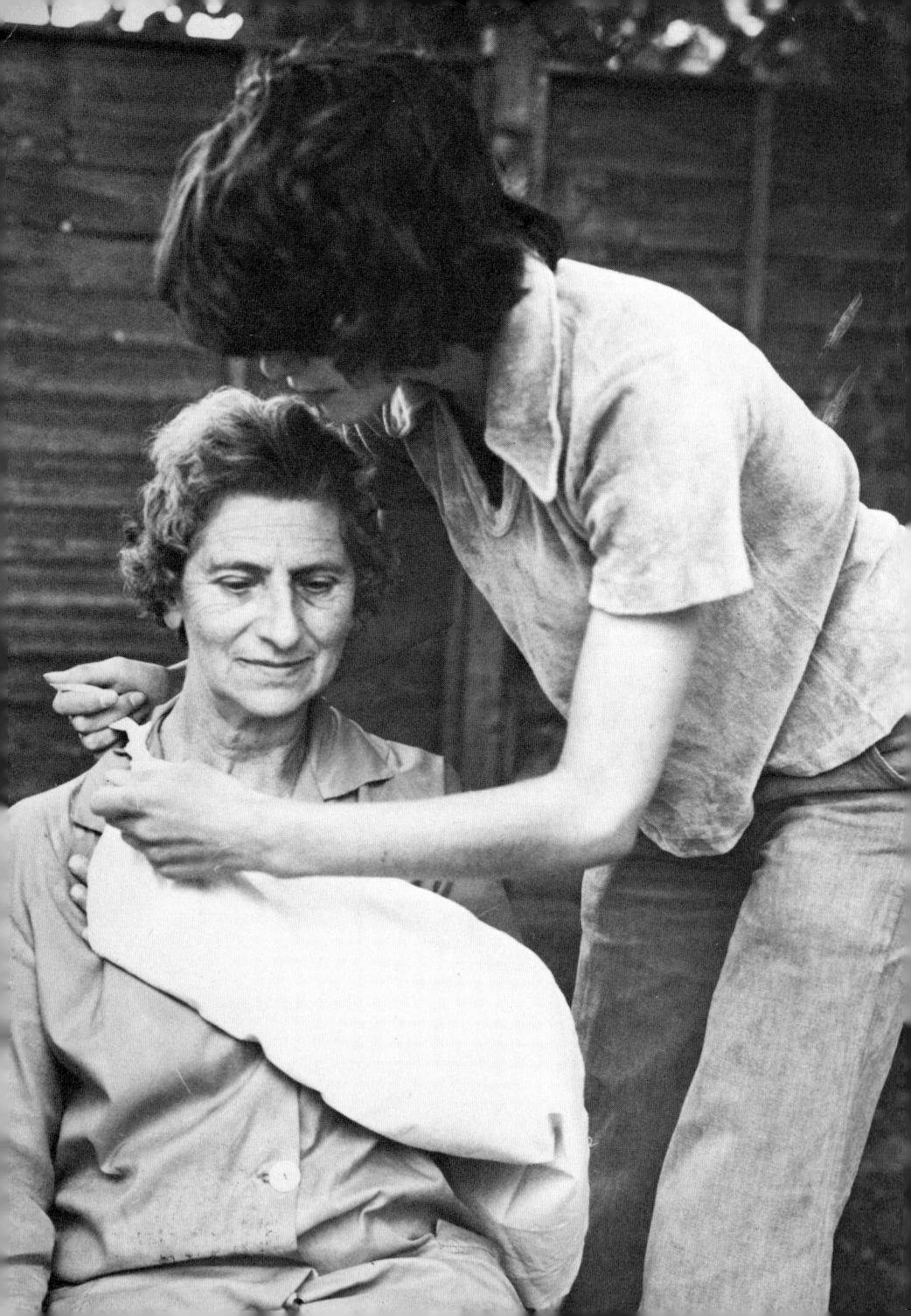

Richard Harrison, MB, FRCS

photographs by Geoff Johnson
and Richard Harrison

FIRST

Illustrated Teach Yourself

AID

KNIGHT BOOKS

Hodder & Stoughton

ISBN 0 340 18489 2

First published in 1976 by Knight Books, the paperback division of Hodder & Stoughton Children's Books, Salisbury Road, Leicester.

Filmset by Keyspools Limited, Golborne, Lancashire.
Printed in Great Britain in Knight Books for Hodder & Stoughton Children's Books, a division of Hodder & Stoughton Ltd, Arlen House, Salisbury Road, Leicester, by Fletcher & Son Ltd, Norwich.

Line illustrations by Susan Hunter

Contents

Quick reference guide for emergencies

1
Life or death: vital priorities in first aid

'If I see an accident, would I know what to do?' You are probably reading this book because you have asked yourself some such question. Perhaps you have already had some instruction in first aid but trained first-aiders are far outnumbered by people who, if pressed, would have to admit that they 'haven't a clue' as to what to do in an emergency. So let us assume that, faced with an individual lying on the ground, and perhaps seriously injured, you would not know how to begin helping him. In ten minutes from now, by the same time it takes to reach the end of this chapter, you will have learnt enough to deal with the really urgent situations and, at least, will be able to keep your patient alive until further help arrives.

The moment you see a casualty – even as you move towards him and kneel down – ask yourself three questions, in this order:

1   Is he likely to suffer any further injury?
2   Is he breathing?
3   Is he bleeding?

If the answers to all three questions are reassuring, you can relax a little. The casualty may be seriously injured, but a few minutes is not going to affect his chances of recovery, and you can tackle the business of diagnosis and treatment in a methodical fashion. Before doing so, let us consider these three vital questions in detail.

The risk, and the correct course of action, may be so obvious as to need no explanation: for example, if the injured person is in a burning house. Sometimes the danger is less evident. Nobody knows how many individuals have been knocked down by one vehicle and, lying in the road, have been killed by another. The difficult decisions are those which have to be made when a danger cannot be assessed exactly. Is the damaged wall beside him going to remain standing, or fall over? And the really dangerous ones, those in which the risk is not perceived – as when a first-aider, kneeling at the roadside on a dark night, does not realise that he, and his patient, are almost invisible to oncoming traffic.

The photographs show various techniques for moving an injured person – but if you are alone, he is heavier than yourself, and only a few yards have to be traversed, gripping his collar and pulling him along on his back, is probably the best method.

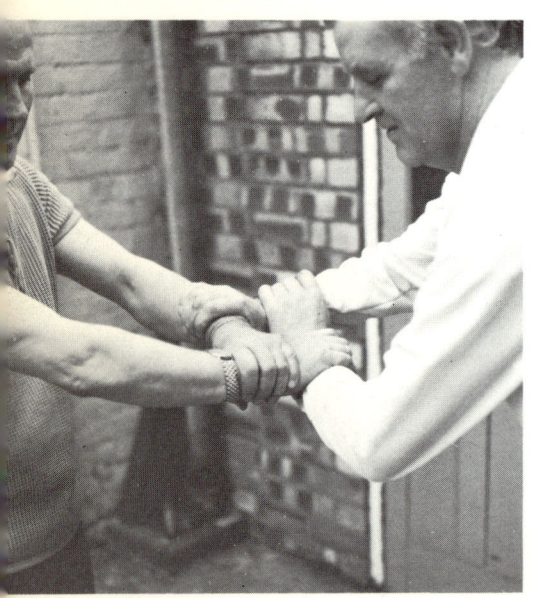
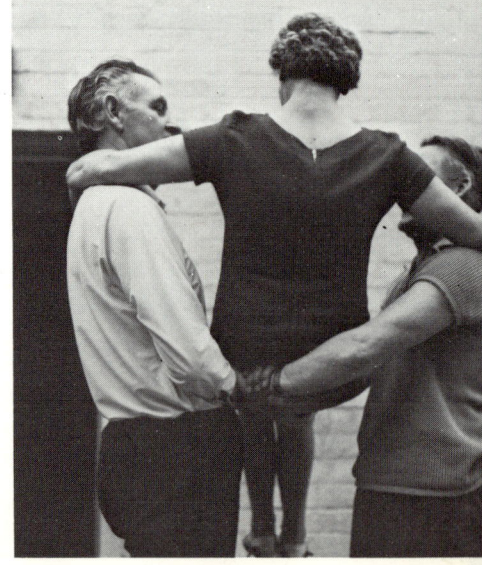

*Techniques for moving a casualty.
Below, left: The two-handed carry.
In an emergency it would be wise
to remove your wrist watch.
Below: The fireman's lift is
useful for carrying an unconscious
patient because the rescuer can
grasp him securely and also have
a free hand; the difficulty is to
get the patient in position.
Right: This single-handed method
is crude and can only be used over
short distances but may be the only
solution in a desperate situation.*

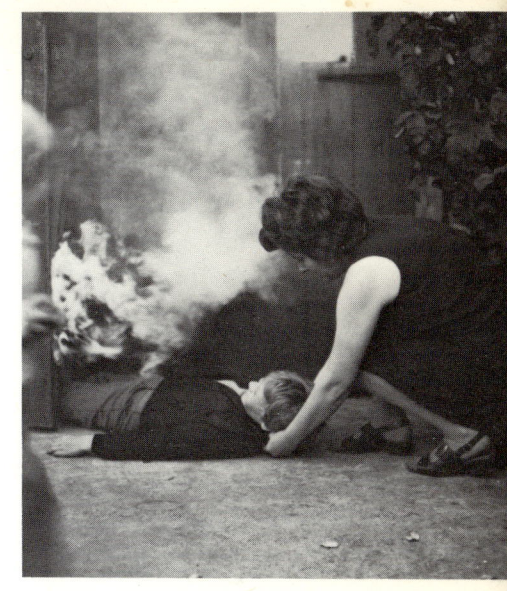

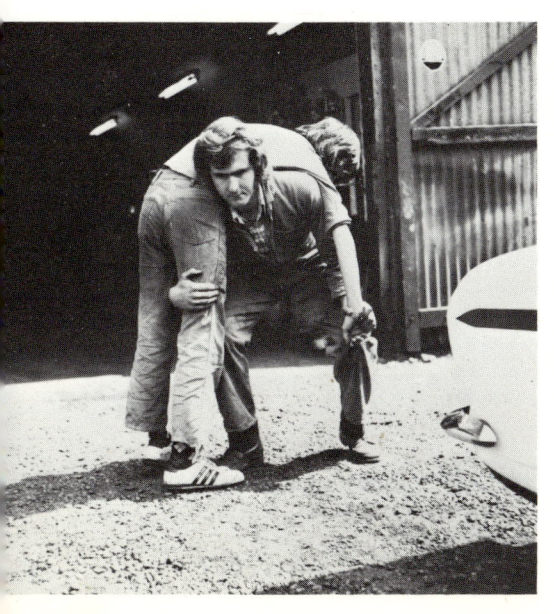

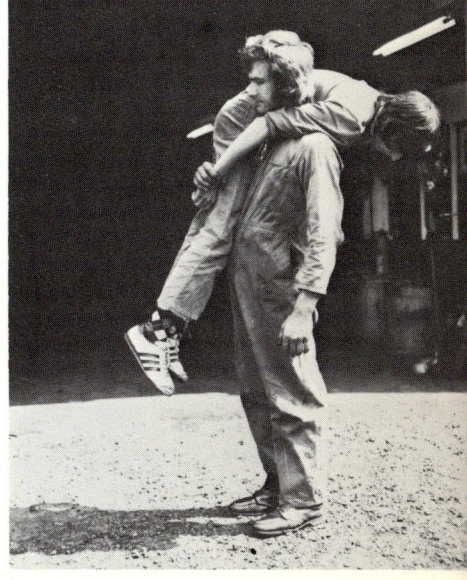

9

IS HE BREATHING?

It is easier to be sure a casualty *is* breathing – that his chest is moving – than to be sure he is not, because quiet, shallow, respiration may be almost undetectable.

The details of artificial respiration are discussed in chapter 6, but even at this stage, the essentials can be outlined.

If in any doubt about whether he is breathing, start artificial respiration and decide later whether you need continue. Turn the subject on his back, whisk your index finger rapidly round his mouth, and as far down the throat as it will easily pass (to remove any obstruction), and then pinch his nostrils between your finger and thumb. Place your mouth across his, and blow hard enough to inflate his chest. Straighten up for a moment, while his chest collapses and you take another breath. Then inflate his chest again and repeat the process for as long as there is a hope that spontaneous breathing will be restored.

IS HE BLEEDING?

If the casualty has an open wound, there will be some loss of blood. During these first few minutes do not worry about a slight oozing, or be too concerned about blood already spilt. Look instead for any wound from which blood is still running, either as a steady trickle, or in spurts. Identify, if there is a large wound and, if you can, the exact part which is bleeding, and place a firm pad over it. A folded handkerchief will do in the first instance. Then, holding that in position with one hand, use your other to take off a tie or belt (your own, or the patient's), with which to fasten the pad in position. The more nearly whatever you use to hold it resembles a broad, flat bandage, wrapped repeatedly round the part to exert a uniform firm pressure, the better it will be: the narrower it is, the less effective. You will now have reduced the rate at which blood is being lost, and can consider the situation more carefully.

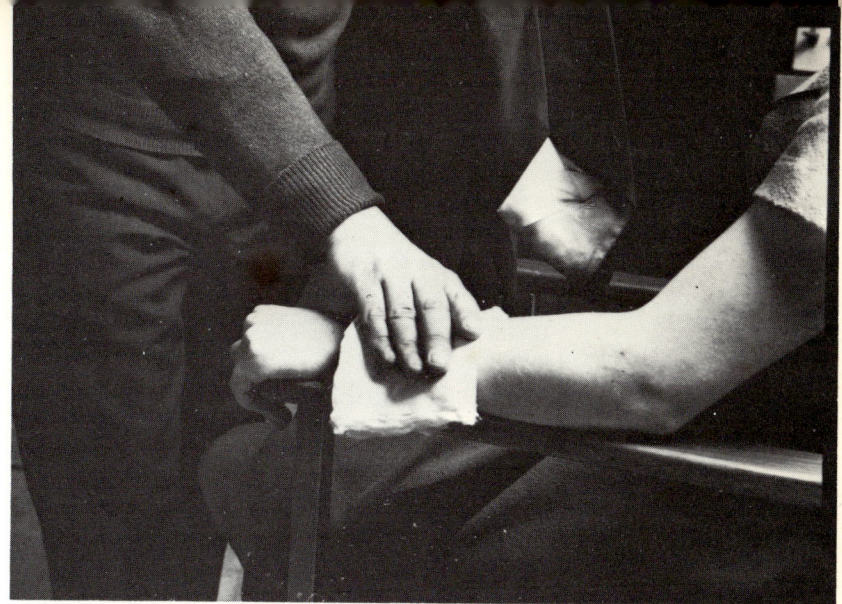

To control a fast-flowing haemorrhage the first aider presses a pad on the wound with one hand and uses the other to tie it in position with an improvised bandage.

MORE THAN ONE CASUALTY

Deciding who to help first can be difficult but there are certain guide-lines. Obviously, someone in imminent danger of sustaining further serious injury (for example, the occupant of a car which is burning, or seems likely to catch fire) must be rescued. A casualty who is completely collapsed, and not breathing, has the second most immediate call for your attention – though there could be circumstances in which his treatment has to stop, because his condition is not improving, and other people are in urgent need of help.

Profuse bleeding from an open wound has the next highest priority and repays attention because it can often be staunched fairly quickly, allowing you to move on and help someone else. When deciding who that is to be, bear in mind that an agitated person who cries repeatedly for assistance, has often sustained less serious injuries than another who lies quietly and makes little complaint.

Anyone who has just been involved in an accident is usually very ready to accept assistance, particularly if they have been injured. Even so, the first-aider should introduce himself, and reassure the casualty in a confident and sympathetic manner. 'I've had to deal with this sort of thing before; we'll soon fix you up' is an appropriate beginning – even if you are wondering what on earth to do next, and how long the ambulance will be! At all costs try to avoid saying, over and over again, some trite phrase. 'I'm a first-aider' is an excellent beginning, but lacks conviction when repeated incessantly for the encouragement of the speaker himself.

Asking what happened sometimes seems superfluous. The sight of an old lady lying at the foot of a staircase may appear to speak for itself. But did she really stumble? Did anyone see the fall? Was it preceded by an epileptic fit? Or has she had a stroke? You may sometimes not have time to take a detailed history, but the omission is always dangerous. The best first-aiders can be recognised by the pains they take to find out exactly what has happened.

It may well be of course, that your patient just cannot provide any history at all, because he or she is unconscious. This is a situation we shall consider in a later chapter, but for the present let us imagine the casualty can talk. Obviously, you will ask him how he was hurt and where his pain is, and will examine first whatever region he indicates.

TAKING THE PULSE

Before doing so, it is a good idea to kneel beside him and take his pulse (see photographs) not just because it is expected of you, but because you thereby discover the state of his circulation. The speed with which the heart is beating, whether its rate is regular or erratic, and the strength of the pulse (that is to say, how easily

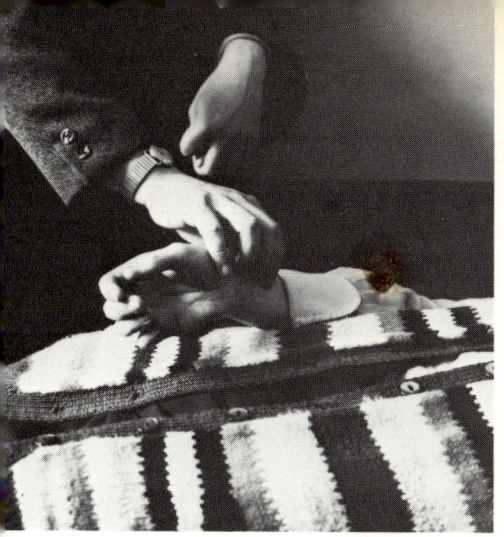
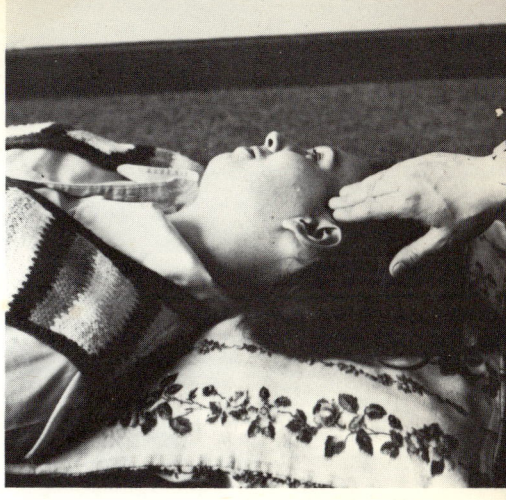

Taking the pulse at the wrist.

When kneeling at the patient's head, the pulse is most easily felt at the temple.

it can be felt) are all valuable pieces of information, but not readily understood by someone unaccustomed to taking a pulse. Even with a little experience though, you will distinguish between the slow, readily detected pulse of a patient who has fainted, and the rapid, almost imperceptible, pulse typical of the very dangerous form of collapse called 'wound shock'.

While feeling for his pulse you also have an excellent opportunity to get back your own breath, consider your next step and – above all – look at the patient's general condition. Is he alert and looking well? Drowsy or unnaturally quiet (as after concussion, or in wound shock)? Flushed or pale (the latter suggesting shock and/or loss of blood)?

Having noted the casualty's overall state, go on to examine the injured region. This raises another problem – how to get at it. As soon as possible after a patient arrives at hospital, the staff remove all or most of his clothes, because accurate diagnosis is impossible without adequate exposure. You are concerned only with an approximate diagnosis and are probably not working in a warm clean room. So expose the injured part as little as possible to avoid the patient becoming chilled, and his wounds dirty, but remove

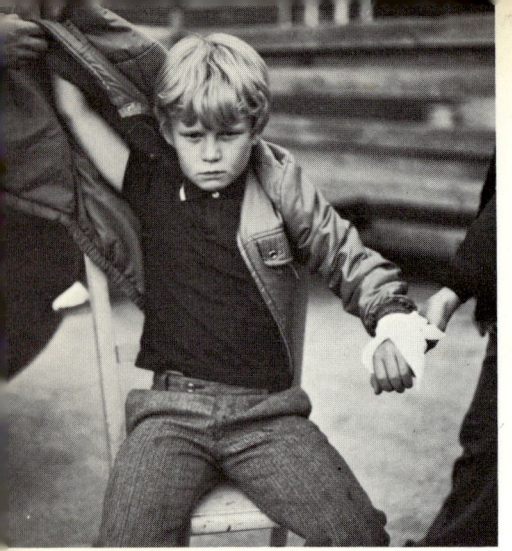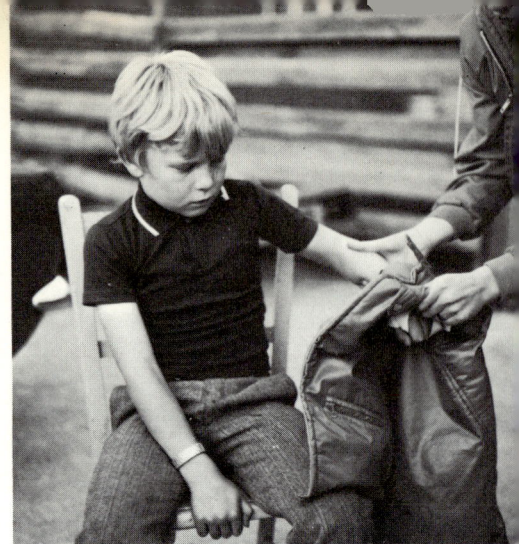

Examining an injury. To take off a patient's coat, pull it from above and behind, and extract an injured arm only when the rest of the garment has been freed.

enough clothing to allow you to inspect the place that is injured. Note whether there is an open wound or bruising, how much bleeding has occurred, and whether the region is swollen or otherwise deformed. Then touch the area gently, to find out if it feels abnormal, or is tender.

Before doing any more, now carry out a rapid, but thorough, survey of the rest of the patient's body. The injury about which a casualty complains may not be his only one and his most obvious wound not necessarily the most serious. Run your hands along the whole length of his body, beginning at the back of the head, and continuing to the finger-tips of first one arm, then the other. As you do so, squeeze the limb gently, and move its joints. While doing this, watch your patient's face (which is a more delicate method of detecting than asking repeatedly 'Am I hurting you'?) Repeat the process with each leg, and then compress the chest a little from side to side, watching to see if you cause any wincing. Then, feel the abdomen and squeeze the crests of the hips together (to detect any damage to the pelvis) as you did in the chest. Finally, feel under the patient, if he is lying on his back, to make sure there is no unsuspected pool of blood beneath him.

This survey can be performed almost as quickly as it has taken you to read about it but in every case, some parts of it — depending on the circumstances of the accident — should be carried out with particular care. Thus, if the individual has fallen from a height, and broken one ankle, it is sensible to examine the other foot carefully and if, in a car smash, a man's head has been bruised and cut, an intelligent first-aider will wonder whether his neck has also been damaged. It is worth reiterating, though, that whenever possible the whole body must be painstakingly examined, simply because every now and again some un-expected, unpredictable, second injury will be found.

Feeling for broken ribs.
The examiner does not lean on his
hands but squeezes them gently.

To detect any damage to the pelvis,
compress the crests of the hips together.

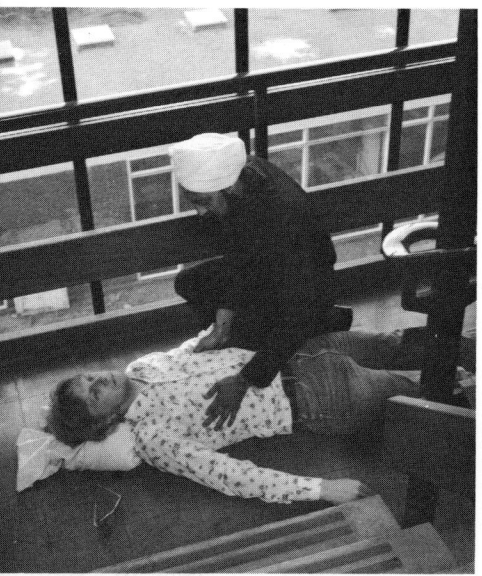

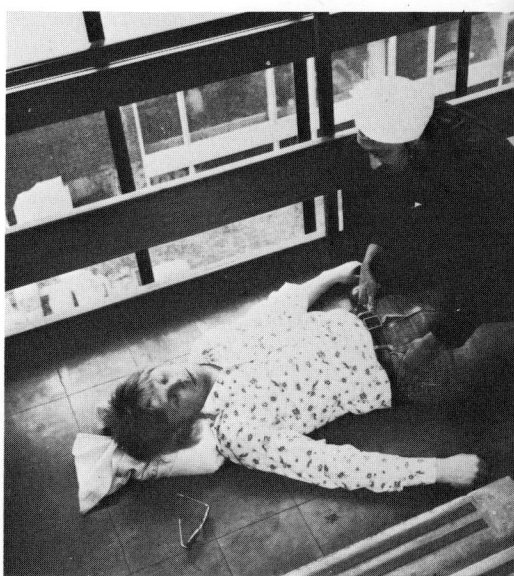

2
A nasty gash: bleeding and how to stop it

THREE SIMPLE STEPS

Later in this chapter we shall consider the different ways in which a person may bleed, and the effects of losing a lot of blood. When coping with a person who is actually bleeding, however, you will feel that it does not matter what sort of blood is coming out or how long it could be before the person collapses! The urgent need is to stop the flow, and here is how to do it:

1   Make the patient rest. If he is excited, or running about, his blood pressure will be raised, and he will bleed that much more fiercely.

2   Raise the bleeding part above the rest of the body. This too, will reduce the 'head of pressure' behind the wound, and

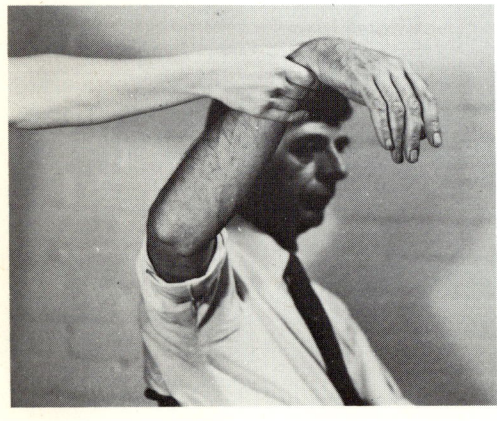

To stop the flow of blood make the patient rest and raise the bleeding part above his head to reduce the head of pressure.

16

slow the rate of loss. So, in the case of a cut on the leg, make the casualty lie on his back and lift his foot on to, for example, a chair. If a hand is injured, make the patient sit down and hold the arm above his head. When the blood is coming from the nose, scalp or face, rest the patient with his head and shoulders elevated.

3   If there is an open wound, place over it the cleanest available soft dressing. (A pad of surgical gauze is ideal but, more often, a folded handkerchief may have to serve.) Press firmly on this and, as soon as you have an opportunity, apply a firm bandage instead of your fingers, to hold the pad in place.

These simple steps will control just about every case of haemorrhage (bleeding) a first-aider is likely to encounter. What if the bleeding does not stop? The emphatic answer is that bleeding from any limb wound can always be controlled by pressure. If it continues, that is because the pressure was too slight, in the wrong place, or not sustained for long enough. Should blood continue to ooze through a dressing, do not take that off. Instead, apply another pad and a firmer bandage over the first.

There are occasions when these steps have to be modified – if the source of bleeding is inaccessible because it is, for example, inside the nose. We shall deal with such situations later.

TYPES OF BLEEDING

An open wound on the surface of the body, such as we have been considering, is the commonest form of haemorrhage. Such a wound, if it is shallow, divides only tiny vessels – those which are, in fact, so small that their diameter is less than that of a hair. For that reason, they are called capillaries after the Latin word (capillus) for a hair. The ordinary, everyday domestic cut sustained, for instance, on the chin while shaving, damages only these, and the bleeding which results needs no description here. Blood reaches capillaries in much larger vessels – arteries –

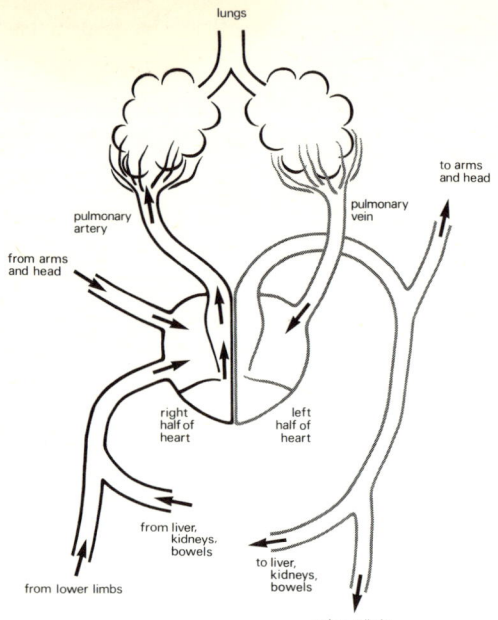

The circulatory system.

which, at their connection with the heart, may be as much as an inch in diameter. They become progressively finer as they run into the limbs and various internal organs, to branch out finally as a network of capillaries.

Should one of the arteries be severed, the bleeding will be profuse and will occur as a series of spurts, corresponding with the casualty's heartbeats. The effect can be very frightening but, in fact, such bleeding, coming from a single, easily identifiable source, is often easier to stop than the less impressive ooze from a wound which has divided many small vessels.

From the capillaries blood flows back to the heart by another network of vessels, which join together and form veins. Most arteries are deep beneath the skin, though their pulsation can be felt at such places as the wrist, and sometimes can be seen in a person's temple. Many veins are deeply situated too, but because several are visible through the skin, we are more familiar with them. When a vein is cut the bleeding, though often profuse, is steady, not spurting and the blood has a darker colour than that from an artery. These distinctions need not concern a first-aider too much. For one thing, a wound which divides a vein often also cuts an artery underneath it, so both types of bleeding result. For another, whether an artery or a vein has been damaged, the remedy is the same – raise the part, and press a pad firmly on to the origin of the haemorrhage.

INTERNAL BLEEDING

There is one form of bleeding which is not spectacular, not easily recognised and sometimes dangerous. If the torn vessels are inside the body – in say, the liver or lungs – the blood may never reach the exterior, or does so only when (depending on its source) it is coughed up, vomited or excreted via the bowel or bladder.

Such bleeding may be suspected if a patient has had a blow on the chest or abdomen, but can occur through disease, and without any history of injury. In either case there will usually be some complaint of pain, but the most striking feature is that the patient collapses, with an increasing pallor of his face and lips. The pulse is difficult to detect, because it is fast and 'thready' (that is the heart tries to compensate for the lack of blood by beating rapidly, but pumps only a small quantity with each stroke). There is often a restless, anxious expression, and a gasping type of breathing – so-called 'air hunger'.

Only in hospital can this type of bleeding be controlled, and the patient should be moved there as a matter of grave urgency. Meanwhile:

a   Keep him as quiet and as calm as possible.
b   Lay him at least flat and, when feasible, raise the legs and the lower part of the trunk higher than his head by tilting the bed, stretcher or plank on which he lies.
c   Lift up his arms, too, if that can be done. The object of these measures is to divert to the most important region, the head, as much of the remaining blood as possible.

SMALL CUTS

The familiar cut from a tin-opener which slips, or from a broken glass, should be washed well. Plenty of warm water (which in Britain is usually almost sterile as it flows from the hot water tap) is less likely to damage the tissues than strong antiseptic solutions. Dry the wound, and then cover it with some gauze or a clean cloth. Bleeding is likely to be troublesome, rather than dangerous, and soon ceases if the limb is elevated above the shoulder, and kept still for five or ten minutes.

Many such trivial cuts do not require medical advice, but that should always be sought if the edges gape – such wounds heal slowly, leave ugly scars and almost inevitably become infected. A stitch or two may save a lot of trouble and pain. Another circumstance which demands an expert opinion is if part of the body beyond the wound is found to be numb, or lacks a normal power of movement. This could be a sign that a nerve or tendon has been damaged, and needs repair.

WOUNDS THAT ARE NOT 'CLEAN'

Wounds with a 'retained foreign body' is the medical term for wounds with extraneous material inside them. Commonly, this material is gravel or particles of dirt. If the 'foreign bodies' are small ones, sticking loosely to the wound, they can be washed away with a gentle stream of water, as described above. They pose a first-aid problem, though, if they are glass or metal, firmly embedded, and the wound is bleeding profusely. Obviously, one cannot, in such cases, stop the bleeding in the way previously described because any pressure on the wound would drive the 'foreign body' in more deeply. Instead, the usual pad has to be fashioned into a ring, which can then be applied round the offending fragments, to press only on the wound edges (see photographs). Do not, in general, try to extract a 'foreign body'

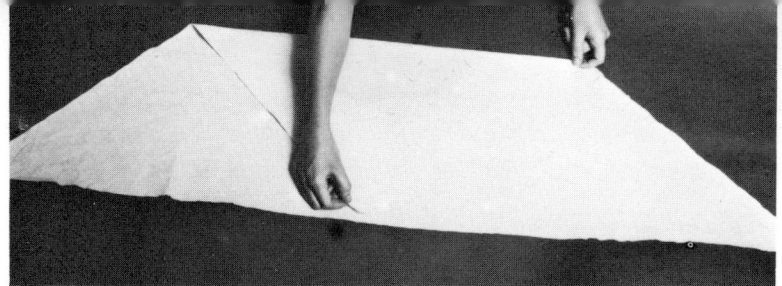

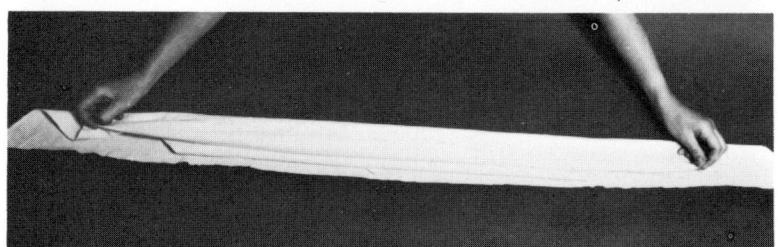

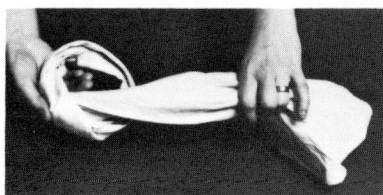

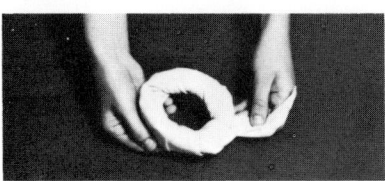

*How to make and apply a ring
bandage for use on 'unclean'
wounds.*

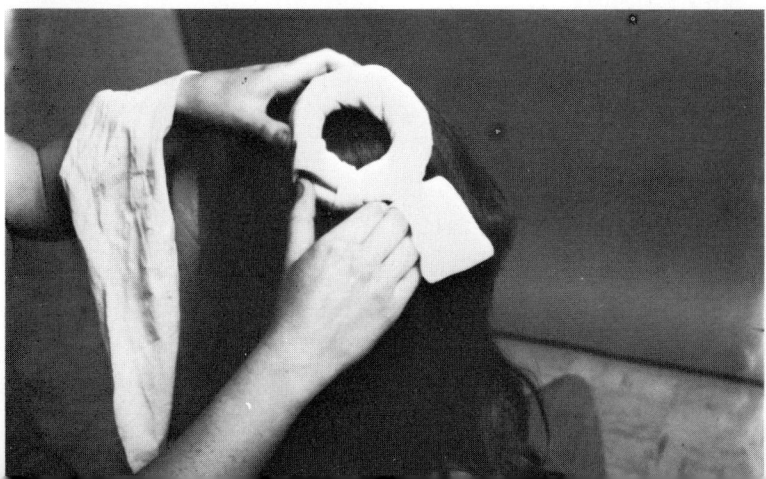

which is not easily removed – there is some risk of causing further bleeding and of damaging nerves or other important structures.

Even if there is little bleeding, and no obvious 'retained foreign body' a doctor should be consulted about any cut which may contain fragments of glass, or which has been contaminated with soil, gravel, wood splinters or anything similar.

PUNCTURE WOUNDS

The holes made by such implements as long, pointed knives, meat skewers and knitting needles are called 'puncture wounds'. Everyone knows these can be very dangerous if the weapon has pierced some vital organ. The patient may then exhibit the signs of internal haemorrhage we have already considered. The wounds themselves, however, do not usually give rise to any first aid difficulties, because they seldom bleed much and look innocuous. Do not be misled by this for it is almost impossible to tell from the appearance of such holes how deep they are, or what damage has been done to internal structures. All such wounds urgently require a doctor's opinion.

We must mention, also, the unusual combination of a puncture wound and a retained foreign body. If you think for a moment, you will realise that this describes a casualty with a knife, or some such object, still sticking in him. The important point to remember is *don't pull it out!* The tip may be plugging the hole it has made in some vital organ; even if it is not, the presence in a wound of the object which made it, helps the doctor to assess how deeply it has penetrated. Only if the wound is already bleeding very dangerously, should this advice be disregarded – for then the knife must be extracted before any pressure can be applied to the wound.

First aid manuals once laid great stress on pressure points. These are the points on the surface of the body where the beating of a large artery can be felt (for instance, the pulse at the wrist), and where the artery, because it runs over a bony surface, can be compressed against it. In dealing with severe haemorrhage from a cut artery, the knowledge of where these points are, and how to compress can be as valuable as knowing where the main stopcock is when a water pipe bursts. The drawback is that they can be difficult to locate – especially if the patient is heavily built or wearing thick clothing – and precious time may be lost trying to find them. For this reason, they are now regarded with less importance than in former years. Two are worth remembering, because they are, as it were, the main stopcocks for the whole arm and the leg respectively.

a   The brachial pressure point (the brachial artery is the principal vessel to the arm). This lies on the inner side of the arm, along a line which more or less coincides with the seam of one's coat.

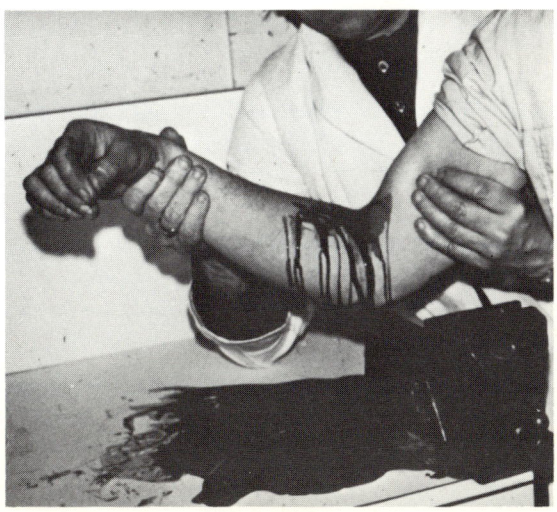

Locating the brachial pressure point.

b The femoral pressure point. This is where the main artery to the leg runs over the upper part of the thigh bone. It is not always easy to identify this but if you span the thigh with both hands, as in the illustration, the tips of your thumbs should be resting on each other and over the artery.

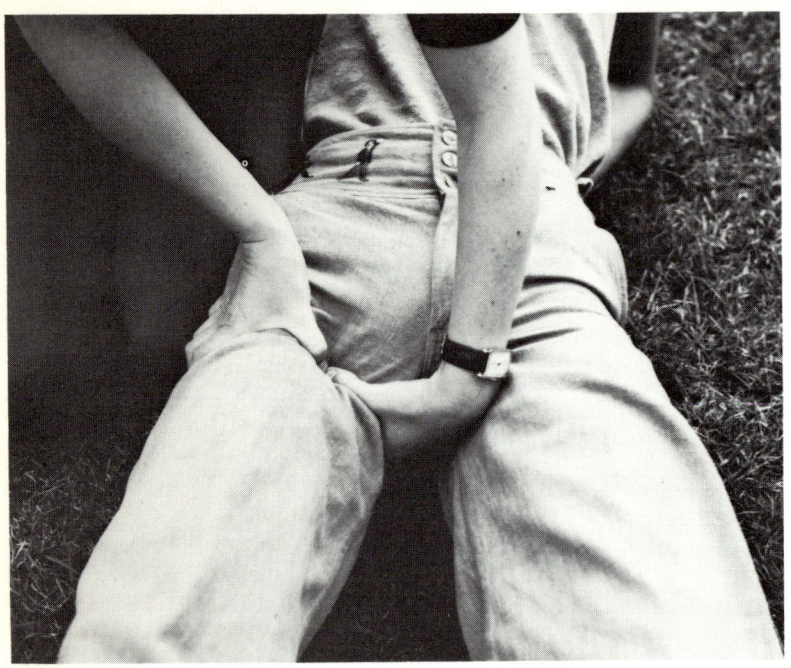

It is not always easy to locate the femoral pressure point.
If you span the thigh with both hands the tips of your thumbs
should rest on each other and on the artery.

By all means familiarise yourself with these two points, by feeling your own arm and thigh and practise, too, stopping haemorrhage from a badly crushed or lacerated hand by placing one thumb on each side of the front of the wrist. Remember, though, that if you ever need to use them, it will be in a rather desperate situation, and perhaps in confused or poorly lit surroundings. You must be able to find them confidently, quickly and without any fumbling.

The subject of tourniquets is no longer mentioned in orthodox first aid manuals but as it crops up sooner or later in all discussions about haemorrhage, we will dispose of it here. A tourniquet is a tight band (classically, of rubber) which, correctly applied round the limb, completely stops the flow of blood into it. This device seems such an excellent one for arresting haemorrhage that you may well wonder why it is now universally condemned for emergency purposes. The answer lies in two words of the definition just cited. When a tourniquet is not correctly applied, it does more harm than good. If, as is commonly the case, it is too loose, it aggravates bleeding by closing the veins, but not the arteries, in which the pressure is higher – so the limb becomes engorged with blood. Every accident surgeon has seen patients brought to hospital, still bleeding from wounds above which a tourniquet has been tied, and which stop bleeding when that is removed! If a tourniquet is too tight, it certainly prevents further haemorrhage, but crushes important nerves and may leave a serious paralysis in its wake.

The other important word in the definition was 'completely', which means just what it implies – and a limb from which the blood supply has been cut off completely begins to die, and will be lost if the tourniquet remains in position for more than an hour or so. The best of all reasons, though, for discarding the tourniquet, is that cases in which bleeding cannot be controlled by the methods already described are very rare indeed.

3
Is it broken? The diagnosis and treatment of fractures

DEFINITIONS

A broken bone is often called a fracture. A fracture is a broken bone. It seems worth saying this, because some people imagine there is a difference – though they are never prepared to say just what it is! Having defined a fracture, let us do the same for two conditions which sometimes closely mimic a broken bone. One is a *dislocation,* in which the ends of two or more bones, meeting to form a joint, are forced apart, out of their normal relationship. The other is a *sprain* – which occurs when the violence to which the joint has been exposed is not sufficient to produce a dislocation but is severe enough to tear some of the ligaments holding the bone ends together.

On occasion it is very difficult, when faced with a painful swelling at the end of a bone, to distinguish between these conditions. Indeed, they may co-exist as when the head of the upper arm bone breaks and is simultaneously dislocated from its socket. Fortunately, this is not a problem which need trouble the first-aider.

WHEN TO SUSPECT A FRACTURE

Everyone knows how most fractures are caused – by some violence being applied to the bone. Occasionally, the bone breaks at the site at which this force acts – a shin bone, kicked hard enough, breaks at the point at which the toe of the boot hits the leg. Individuals knocked down while crossing the road often suffer a fracture of one or other of the leg bones at exactly the level at which the vehicle's bumper struck them. Fractures produced in this way, by direct violence, are not nearly so common as those in which a whole limb, or some other region of the body, has been exposed to violence, and has given way at its weakest part. Thus, many fractures are due to falls but, when we stumble and drop on to our hands and knees, we do not break our knee caps and our fingers. Instead, the bones near the ankles suffer, because they have been violently twisted, and the shock from the hand hitting the ground is transmitted to the forearm, which buckles under the strain.

In the case of a healthy young adult, considerable force is required to break a bone; the skeleton of a child is more delicate and will crack under lesser degrees of violence; that of an old person is very brittle, and often gives way under a strain which would have no effect on a younger person.

From this you will appreciate that almost any blow or fall can, on occasion, cause a fracture, and the first-aider must always be alert to this possibility. Sometimes the diagnosis is obvious:

a   If the skin has been torn, and the ends of the broken bone are actually visible.

(This is called an open fracture or, using a rather old-fashioned term, a compound fracture.) There is no simpler diagnosis in the whole of first aid than a severe open fracture. Sometimes the skin wound is no more than a small hole,

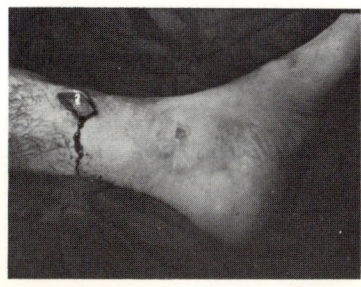

The open fracture may cause only a small skin wound.

which usually oozes blood rather freely: sometimes a skin wound – particularly on a finger – will expose part of a bone which is, in fact, unbroken.

b   If there is a striking deformity.
This may be an unnatural angle in an arm or leg, or a dent on the surface of the chest or head. Very often there is an open wound, as in an open fracture and, even when the skin has not been torn, the sharp bone ends can be seen and felt, because it is stretched over them.

Other deformities are not quite obviously due to a fracture, but can be instantly recognised by a first-aider who has seen or read about them previously – such as the 'dinner fork' deformity of the commonest fracture of the forearm (Colles fracture: see page 65), or the way in which the leg twists and the foot falls sideways, when the upper end of the thigh bone has snapped.

Not every gross, painful deformity is due to a fracture. A dislocated hip can closely resemble the fracture just mentioned, and the most skilled surgeon cannot always distinguish between an ankle which is broken, and one which has been severely sprained. Such distinctions have little bearing on first aid, since the initial treatment of all such injuries is the same.

c   If the bone ends can be felt, or heard, moving against each other.
When one fragment touches another, a very characteristic grating or clicking occurs, which is more easily felt by the hand than heard through the ear. The phenomenon is distinctly uncommon, because usually movement between the bone ends is either restricted by swelling of the tissues, or because they have been jammed together or 'impacted'. The casualty, too, tries to avoid any movement which might produce it, because of the accompanying pain and no one with any knowledge of first aid tries to produce it deliberately. There are occasions though when, while a limb is

being handled or moved, this *crepitus,* as it is called, is felt. Then the diagnosis is established without doubt.

Fortunately, very many fractures are not severe enough to give rise to any of these signs. Often they entail no more than a crack in the bone. In such cases the patient complains of pain, and may not be able to use the limb but, on examining the part, the only obvious signs of injury are those which are also seen when the tissues have been merely bruised or sprained. That is to say they are swollen, tender and discoloured.

What is to be done if the diagnosis is doubtful? Consider the possible courses of action:

a   If the bone is broken, and is treated correctly, the patient will be spared further pain and the fracture will get no worse.

b   If the bone is broken, but the patient is urged to go on using the limb, he will suffer increasing discomfort and the bone ends may shift, aggravating the damage.

c   If the bone is not broken, but is treated as if it were – well, the patient has had more care and attention than he may have deserved, but he will probably be relieved and no harm has been done.

The correct approach to the problem is obvious – when in doubt, suspect a bone is broken and proceed as if it were.

TREATMENT

Immobilise the fracture–and do it as soon, and as firmly, as possible. Later in this chapter some common fractures, and the best ways of fastening each are considered in detail. Very many different ways of splinting broken bones have been devised, but most have the drawback of needing special equipment or many bandages. In an emergency you may have no more than the clothes you are wearing and, perhaps, the handkerchief in your pocket. Here are some simple measures which can be applied in any situation:

If you have only two bandages (or a tie and a handkerchief) apply one as a figure-of-eight round both ankles, and with the other fasten the knees together.

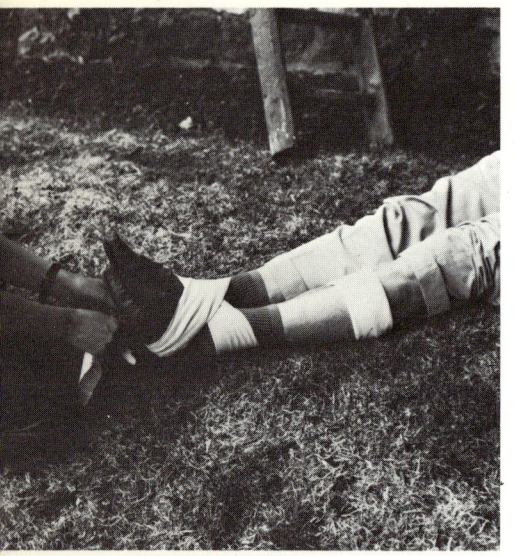
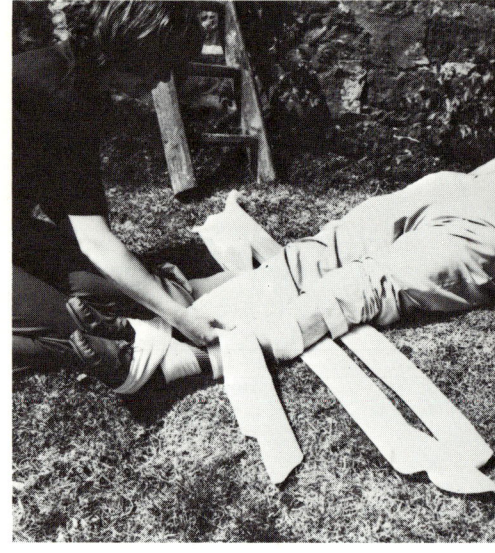

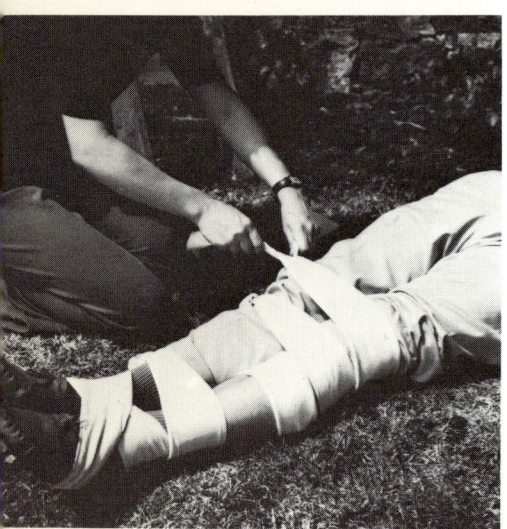

For fractures in the lower limb the figure-of-eight bandage is very important: it ties the patient's feet together and prevents the damaged limb slipping back into deformity. Ideally the bandage should tie on the side of one or other shoe.

If you can find two extra bandages (or can take a belt, and tie or handkerchief, off the patient) pass these round both limbs one above and one below the fracture. Depending on the circumstances, you may need to use one bandage to fasten the cleanest available dressing over a wound (if the fracture is of the open variety), and you may be able to achieve a more secure result by padding the gaps between the patient's legs and ankles with any soft material you can find – for example, a rolled-up towel, cardigan or sweater.

The most important single bandage is the figure-of-eight, tying together the feet. It can also be the most difficult to adjust, if the broken limb is twisted, or at an awkward angle. Study the position of the leg, as you first find it. Kneel at the patient's feet, then grasp the one on the injured side. Draw the limb down with a firm steady motion (not a sudden pull, or a series of jerks!) and align it with the undamaged one. Someone else may now tie the bandage for you, or you can hold the patient's heels between your knees. At all costs, avoid letting the broken limb roll over sideways or slip back into deformity, once you have corrected its position.

FRACTURES IN THE UPPER LIMB

If the break is above the elbow, that part of the arm can be bandaged to the patient's side, and then a sling applied to support the forearm. Only three bandages are required. Two are applied respectively above and below the suspected fracture, and the third is used for the sling. The usual difficulty lies not in obtaining these bandages, but in finding enough padding to make a comfortable, firm job of the immobilisation – and this is a problem which varies with the build and sex of the patient.

When the forearm is fractured, some form of separate, rigid splint is almost essential. Fortunately only a very short one is required, and a magazine or a stout twig serves very well. If a newspaper or magazine is being used, it can be formed into a trough, inside which the limb rests; or a piece of wood may be placed in front of the limb, and tied to it with whatever bandages can be contrived. Then the arm and splint are supported together in the sling.

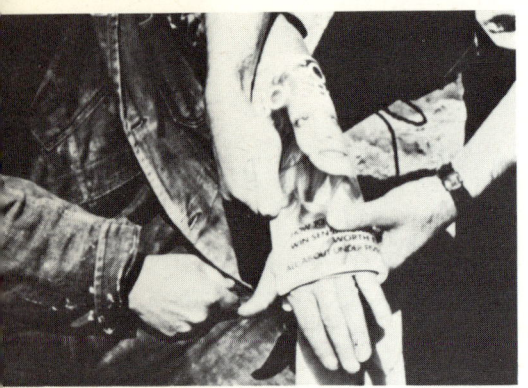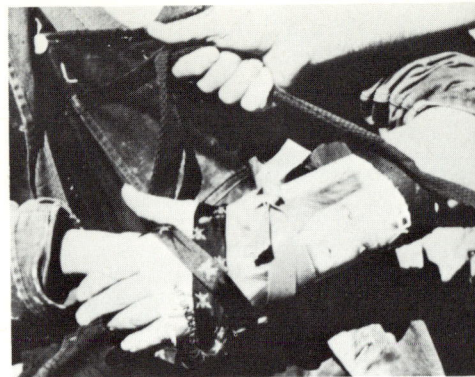

A rigid splint is essential for fractures of the forearm. The arm may rest in a trough formed from a magazine, tied to it by improvised bandages.

SOME SPECIAL FRACTURES

When the broken bone is at the very end of a limb – say, at the shoulder or in the foot – the foregoing advice needs some modification, and this is also true of fractures in the head or trunk. Some of these situations are described below but fractures of the skull are considered in chapter 5.

FRACTURES AT THE SHOULDER

It is very unusual for the shoulder blade to break but three other injuries occur in the same region. The upper end of the humerus (the arm bone above the elbow) may break, or come out of its joint with the shoulder blade – it is not easy to distinguish between the two conditions and the application of a sling is an appropriate treatment for both. Commoner than either injury, however, is a broken collar bone. This is easily diagnosed, because the bone lies so close to the surface that the site of the patient's pain can be

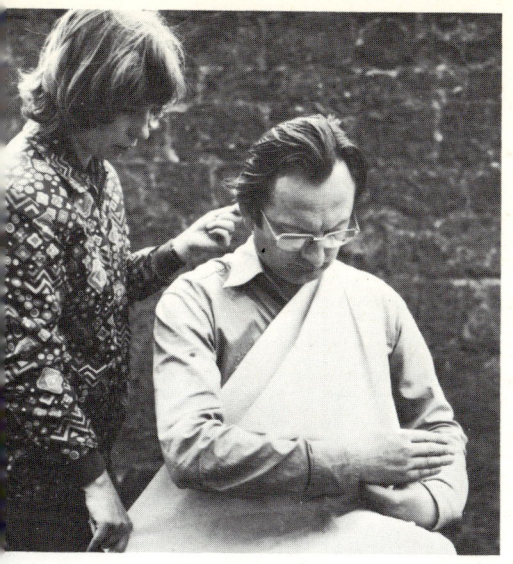
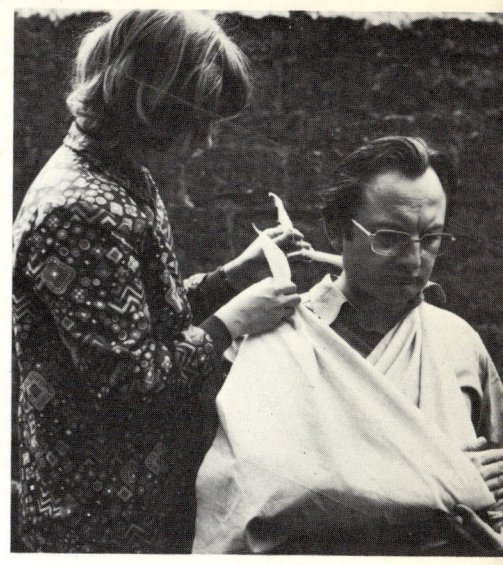

Three stages in the making of an ordinary sling used for fractures at the shoulder.

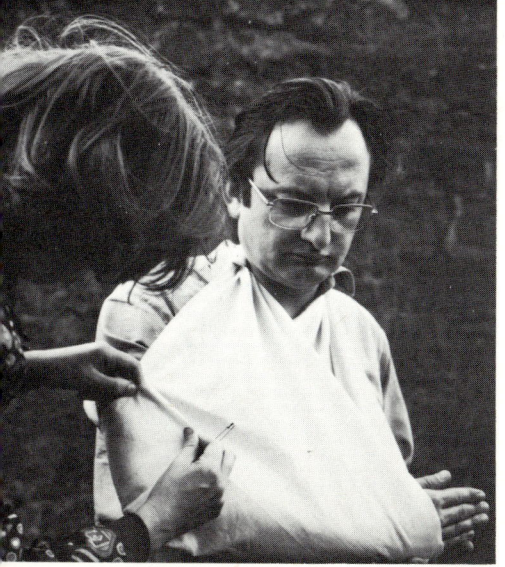

very accurately localised. Often the diagnosis can be made before the patient is examined – from the touchline if the injury is sustained, as it frequently is, during a game of rugby. This is because the manner in which he uses his sound limb to support the other is so very characteristic. An ordinary sling is appropriate, but the 'St John's' style is even better. (See photographs.)

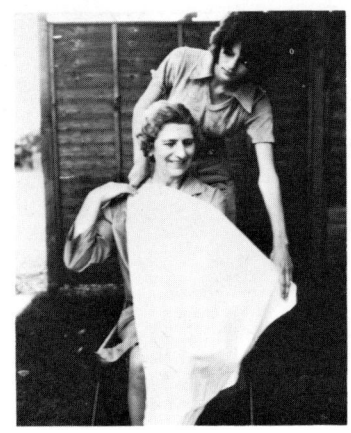 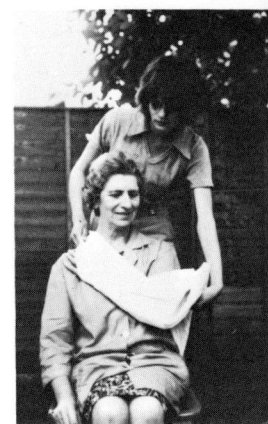

FRACTURES ROUND THE HIP

A broken hip, and a dislocation there, are easily confused, as at the shoulder. Again, the same treatment suffices for both injuries, the limbs in this case being tied together with, if possible, a firm broad bandage (for example, a scarf) wound round the hips for extra support.

Fractures of the pelvis are common, very varied as regards their principal features and the way in which they occur, and sometimes difficult to recognise. Often they are the result of a heavy fall sideways, but others are caused by 'run over' accidents, or by the patient dropping on to his feet from a considerable height and shearing part of the bone. There is usually no obvious deformity but walking or any other movement of the lower part of the trunk is painful, as is even gentle compression of the two hips. Tie the legs together and restore the stability of the damaged bone as much as possible by several bandages, passed under the buttocks and round the hips, and broad enough to overlap each other.

The St John's style sling shown in five stages.

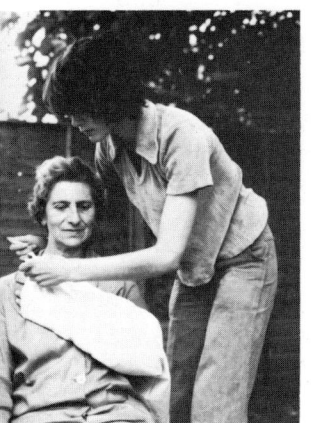 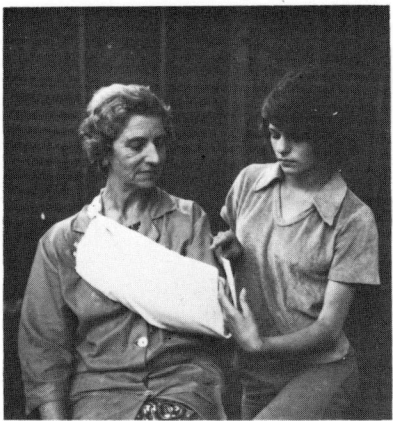 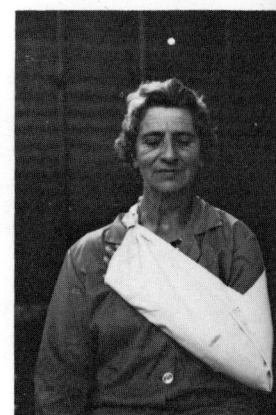

BROKEN FINGERS AND TOES

Elaborate splints, or even the fastening together of adjacent fingers or toes, are unnecessary. The tendons and the other bones of the hand or foot will ensure reasonable immobilisation – unless the injury is gross. A soft, spongy dressing helps to control swelling and makes the part less painful. The ideal materials are a roll of fluffed-out surgical gauze and a crepe bandage; in an emergency one of dry grass and a big handkerchief may be the best available substitutes.

The soft padding is placed in the palm and the fingers are bent gently over it: do not place them in a tightly clenched position. If the quantity and nature of the padding is appropriate, arrange some of it between the individual fingers and over the back of the hand. Then apply the bandage so that the injured hand is in the centre of a cocoon, under just enough pressure to stop any bleeding and immobilise the broken bones. In the case of the foot, the whole of it or, if only the toes are damaged, those and the forefoot alone, can be wrapped inside a firm, compact bundle.

35

Contrary to popular belief, these fractures are neither very rare nor, for the most part, particularly disabling. The spine or 'backbone' is not a single entity, but is composed of some two dozen individual members – the vertebrae – joined together by strong ligaments. It is most often injured by forces which tend to compress this chain of linked bones from end to end – by a fall in which the victim sits down heavily, or strikes the ground feet first. When this happens one or more of the vertebrae, usually those in the small of the back, are likely to be crushed.

Because the ligaments remain intact, and the integrity of the chain as a whole does not suffer, the symptoms of such fractures are often only pain and stiffness in the region affected. Sometimes, particularly if he sustains other and more distressing injuries in the same fall, the individual remains unaware of the damage to his back, which requires X-ray films for its diagnosis. The first-aider who is consulted by a patient who complains of backache some hours or days after a fall, can do no more than suspect what has happened, and advise further investigation. Serious long-term effects are unusual.

There is a second type of fracture which is very different. This usually results from violence which tends to shear, instead of compressing, the chain of vertebrae, as when the spine is violently flexed by a weight dropping on a man's shoulders while he is stooping down. The bony damage to one or more vertebrae (at whatever level the violence acts) is less important than the fact that they may shift on each other and, in doing so, injure the spinal cord or the nerves from it, which run through these bones and are normally protected by them.

The patient is aware of severe pain and a sense of instability in his back. If there is any nerve damage he also loses sensation and the power of movement, below the level of the fracture. Treatment must be such as will not aggravate the nerve damage by causing any further shifting of the unstable vertebrae.

1   Faced by a casualty who is lying on the ground after a serious fall or blow which has caused pain in his back, leave him where he is until a doctor arrives, if possible.

2   If he has to be moved, try to transport him *in the same position* in which he has been lying. Someone lying on his face is carried face downwards; on his back, face upwards.

3   If he is carried by hand, with someone at his shoulders and someone else holding his legs, he is emphatically not being kept *in the same position,* for his spine will sag between the bearers. So summon several helpers (six are ideal) and lift the casualty very carefully on to something which will serve as a stretcher. Sagging as he is raised, will be minimised if those holding the head and legs pull slightly against each other, to keep the backbone straight.

4   If a proper stretcher is not available, commandeer a door or gate.

RIB INJURIES

Two types of rib fracture may be encountered by the first-aider.

a   If the patient has broken only one or two ribs and their ends are not displaced, his general condition is likely to be good, even though he may complain of severe pain. Gentle pressure down one or other side of his chest discloses the site of the injury (because ribs comparatively seldom break at the back, or in the front). A bandage which constricts his chest may relieve him, but lying him down with the trunk inclined towards the damaged side is often even more effective. Fractures of this type are often the result of a fall in which some such object as a post, or the corner of a box, has struck the chest.

b   Fractures which involve several ribs are much more dangerous and, fortunately, less common. The violence of a road accident can produce such injuries, in which the ribs are not only broken but displaced, so that the chest is deformed and breathing is seriously impaired. Bandaging is less effective here. Any open wound must be covered as quickly as possible by a bulky pad, to make a dressing which is as nearly airtight as possible. The patient's posture should be arranged to assist his respiration (usually, by raising his shoulders and turning him slightly towards the injured side). Treat him for shock (see below) and move him to hospital as quickly and as gently as possible.

SHOCK

Finally, it must be stressed that many fractures are complicated by a general collapse of the patient. This is due to wound shock which is described in the next chapter and the first-aider must do what he can to anticipate and reduce this. He must also bear in mind, though, that when the patient reaches hospital it may be necessary to give a general anaesthetic when the broken bone is re-aligned and placed in plaster. It helps the anaesthetist if the patient has an empty stomach, so the traditional 'cup of hot sweet tea' is best omitted.

4
Shock: the potential killer

If an individual receives extensive injuries – for instance, a fracture across both thigh bones – he may die during the next twenty-four hours. This fact causes no undue surprise – but it should do so, because there is nothing inevitably fatal about breaking two bones, even if they are the biggest in the body. In many instances, the killer is the condition called 'shock'.

'A SHOCK'

It is not well named, for the word 'shock' has confused first-aiders ever since it was introduced in this particular connection, a hundred and thirty years ago. We tend to associate the term with the sense in which it is used in everyday life – meaning the emotional upset, and sometimes the physical faintness, which follows an unpleasant surprise. This confusion is increased by the fact that even minor injuries are sometimes followed by a collapse which has much in common with what the ordinary person calls 'a shock' – for instance, the man or woman who turns pale immediately after cutting a finger-tip, and needs to sit down. Such faintness is usually brief, requires no special treatment and is followed by spontaneous recovery.

SHOCK

What we are concerned with here is entirely different, and it is a pity that this condition is not designated by some special medical name which would be less ambiguous. It is sometimes referred to as 'wound shock': in this book, however, we shall call it simply 'shock'.

The exact nature and cause of this dangerous collapse which follows injury are not known, despite an immense amount of medical research into the subject, but a typical case is easily recognised. The casualty has always sustained a serious injury – and if shock (true shock, not the passing pallor and faintness mentioned above) begins to develop in someone who does not *seem* badly hurt, another unsuspected injury must be looked for. The phrase 'a serious injury' means, however, an injury which is serious for the patient concerned: small children or elderly people are liable to become shocked after wounds which cause comparatively little upset in a healthy adult.

APPEARANCE OF SHOCK

A period of well-being occurs immediately after wounding. The casualty may talk and joke with those helping him for as long as half an hour. During this time his body is making adjustments to compensate for various effects of his injury and, particularly, for any loss of blood. Then a point is reached at which no further adjustment is possible – and the patient, quite suddenly, over perhaps five or ten minutes, becomes quiet. He makes very little spontaneous movement, and grows pale. Small beads of perspiration appear on his face, but his skin is cold to the touch. His breathing usually becomes shallower but instead, may have a gasping character. His pulse is so faint and rapid that it is difficult to count. Some faculties, however, are not lost: the patient can hear, though his vision may be poor and he commonly closes his eyes. He will reply to questions, is conscious and sometimes very alert until he lapses into an unconsciousness which is quickly followed by death.

WHAT CAUSES IT?

As has been said, the reason for this collapse is not clear, but many of its features can be explained if we suppose that the volume of blood in the body becomes insufficient to fill the system through which it is normally being pumped – either because blood has been lost by haemorrhage or because, instead of some blood vessels being closed while others are open, all the body's vessels dilate simultaneously.

It is much easier to prevent shock than it is to correct it after it has appeared. A patient who has developed the typical rapid pulse, low blood pressure and pale clammy features may recover spontaneously, or may need a great deal of treatment to save his life, but the process takes several hours. It is comparatively easy to prevent him 'going into shock' but, to do this, the onset of the condition must be foreseen.

WHEN IS IT LIKELY TO OCCUR?

Experience has shown that shock inevitably follows any severe injury – when one or more large bones have been broken, or a great deal of soft tissue has been torn or crushed. It is more marked after a very painful injury than one involving a less sensitive part of the body; wounds associated with the loss of much blood are particularly likely to cause severe shock.

In this connection, it is important to realise that blood can be 'lost' without any obvious haemorrhage. When a thigh bone is fractured, two or three pints of blood may escape into the muscles round it. Unless the fracture is an open one, there will be no external bleeding but the blood will have escaped from the circulatory system and been lost as effectively as if it had been spilled on the pavement. Another point is that the volume of blood circulating will be reduced if its fluid part escapes, even though the red pigment is left behind – such as occurs with the oozing and blistering of widespread burns.

. Just as some types of injury are particularly likely to cause shock, so some types of patient are particularly susceptible. Shock will develop less quickly, and less severely, in a strong healthy man than in a more feeble person – so one has to be very much on the look out for it in children, old people, and those in poor physical condition. Fatigue, thirst and hunger all aggravate its effects and so, too, can worry or mental depression. A military surgeon summed up these latter factors very neatly when he said 'In a retreat shock is more common, and more severe than during an advance'.

TREATMENT

When really severe shock has developed, the only effective treatment is to 'top up', the depleted circulatory system and replace the fluid which has been lost by external haemorrhage, or by oozing into the tissues or into vessels which are more dilated than they should be. This usually means blood transfusion.

There are, however, several very valuable measures a first-aider can take which will delay or minimise the development of shock:

1 Obviously the loss of any more blood must be stopped as soon as possible.

2 The circulation to the most important part of the body, the brain, must be maintained, even if it is failing elsewhere. This is done by placing the casualty with his head lower than his feet.

3 The amount of pain must be reduced not only for simple humanitarian reasons but also because pain and, particularly, the discomfort associated with movement have been shown, over and over again, to aggravate shock.

4 The casualty must be warmed – *but only to a certain extent*. Though a shocked person looks cold and his skin is clammy to the touch, this is seen as a sign that his body is compensating for a failing circulation by shutting down non-essential vessels on the body surface. Heating him may by-pass this process and improve the colour of his skin but, at the same time, blood is diverted from vital internal organs and so his overall condition worsens. If, on the other hand, the person's

42

temperature falls too far, he may begin to shiver and this could be disastrous (shivering is a form of exertion and uses up energy). He must be warmed only enough to prevent this from happening.

There remains one other traditional treatment to be discussed – the celebrated 'cup of warm, sweet tea'. This is, of course, a source of heat, energy and fluid but against this must be set the fact that it often causes vomiting, depleting the body's supply of fluid still further; if an anaesthetic is given even several hours later, the tea may be vomited then, causing breathing difficulties. Certainly, neither tea, nor any other fluid, should be given if there is any suspicion of internal injury.

There may still be a place for this old-fashioned remedy but only in rather unusual circumstances – for instance, if a casualty has sustained injuries only to his limbs and there is no likelihood of his receiving a general anaesthetic for a long time. Its real role though, is as a domestic treatment for minor injuries causing not true shock but 'a shock' such as we discussed at the beginning of this chapter. Its effect then depends, not upon its warmth or sweetness but upon the sedative and restorative action ordinarily attributed to 'a nice cup of tea'.

A SUMMARY

Perhaps after reading this chapter, you feel you do not fully understand the condition of shock. If so, you are not alone – research workers have been puzzling over it for more than seventy years. Here, in summary, are the proven facts which all first-aiders must know.

Shock is a state of general collapse which follows some injuries. It is particularly likely if:

the wound bleeds or oozes a lot;
is very painful;
crushes or damages much tissue.

the patient	is very old or young;
	is in bad health or poor condition;
	is exhausted or depressed.

the characteristic features are

a pale, ashen complexion;
a thin, rapid pulse;
shallow, feeble breathing.

| NOT | noisy, agitated behaviour (though sometimes a certain restlessness is seen); |
| | loss of consciousness (the mind of a shocked patient is usually quite clear until his condition becomes very grave indeed). |

The best treatment is prevention:
1 stop any bleeding
2 avoid moving the patient more than is absolutely essential
3 spare him pain, by bandaging and/or splinting his injuries
4 put his head down or his legs up
5 do not let him shiver.

5
A bang on the head and other causes of unconsciousness

For most of us, there is something peculiarly un-nerving about the sight of a senseless individual. This is due in part to doubt and apprehension. Is he about to open his eyes, or is he on the point of death? In part, it comes from a feeling of helplessness and frustration at being unable to help someone who is very obviously in trouble. In fact, there are certain steps which should be taken immediately when dealing with an unconscious patient, and which may make all the difference to his survival.

a   Make sure he is in no danger of sustaining a fresh injury – for instance, that he will not be hurt if he should suffer some fit or convulsion. Protect his head and trunk, if they are resting on hard or sharp surfaces.

b   Confirm there is no external obstruction to his breathing. Loosen any tight constriction about the neck.

c   Relieve, as much as is possible, any internal obstruction. Noisy respiration, and purple congested features, suggest the windpipe is blocked by mucus, or some other material which has been inhaled. A first-aider may not be able to clear such an obstruction completely but running a finger inside the mouth will detect something like a displaced denture. Pulling the patient's chin forwards, and bending the head backwards, often makes a surprising difference to the way in which he is breathing.

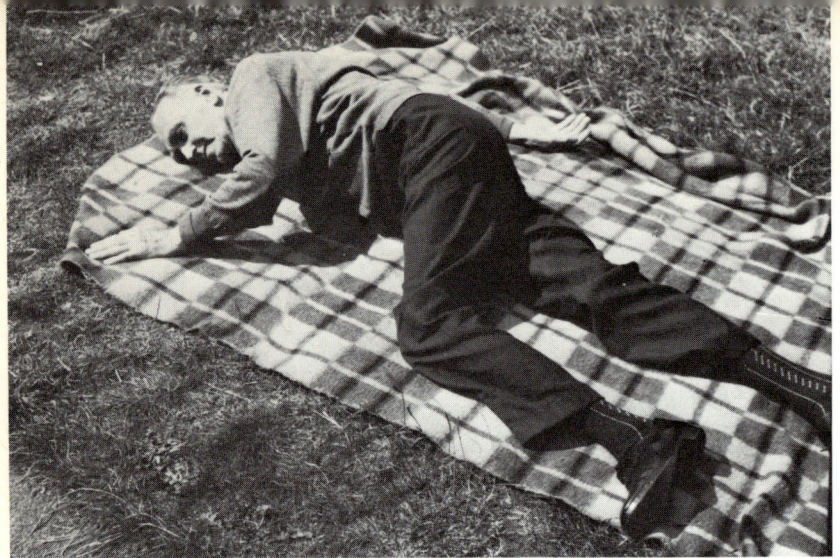

*The recovery position for an unconscious patient
which allows him to breathe easily*

d Position him in such a way that he will continue breathing
easily, and so that if his mouth fills with vomit, saliva or
mucus it will drain away, and not be inhaled to cause further
obstruction. The recommended posture is one in which he
lies on one side, rolled partly on to his face, with one arm and
leg bent up to hold him there. (See photograph.)

COMMON CAUSES OF UNCONSCIOUSNESS

Having taken these precautions, one can set about trying to
discover why consciousness was lost. A list of all the possible
causes would fill a much larger book than this but only half a
dozen occur frequently. If you are called to an individual lying
senseless in the street in this country, the probability is that he
has:
a sustained a head injury, or
b had an epileptic fit, or
c taken drugs or alcohol.

46

Less likely causes for his condition are some disease such as diabetes, or a stroke; he may have fainted, or even been having an acute hysterical seizure. How can we distinguish between these?

A head injury is often suggested by the circumstances in which the casualty is found, and confirmed by visible or obvious signs of damage. Look not only for any swelling or depression on the skull, but also for fluid (clear or bloodstained) running from the ears – a sign of a crack in the floor of the skull, which communicates with the interior of the ear.

If the injury is a relatively mild one, consciousness returns quickly but the patient is often confused, and must on no account be left to his own devices. Any head injury which causes a loss of consciousness, however brief, can be followed by a dangerous relapse and demands a doctor's advice. Any external wound, or discharge from the ears, is meanwhile treated simply by ordinary dressings and bandages.

Epileptic fits are seen less often nowadays but no one who has witnessed a typical attack has any difficulty in recognising another.

The patient may suddenly cry out, then fall down and make a series of convulsive movements with some or all of his limbs. His face becomes blue and congested, and he may literally foam at the mouth. If the churning motion of his jaws damages his lips or tongue, this foam becomes bloodstained. During a severe fit, the person is so helpless that he may suffer much more serious injuries – as from falling into an open fire; very commonly he soils his clothing through losing control of his bladder and bowels.

While the fit lasts, the first-aider can do no more than make sure the patient does not hurt himself, and can breathe freely. Prevent him in particular, from banging his head or biting his tongue. The latter is more easily said than done. The end of a pen, a teaspoon, or similar object should be eased between his jaws but bear in mind that it is not much use protecting the tongue if one or

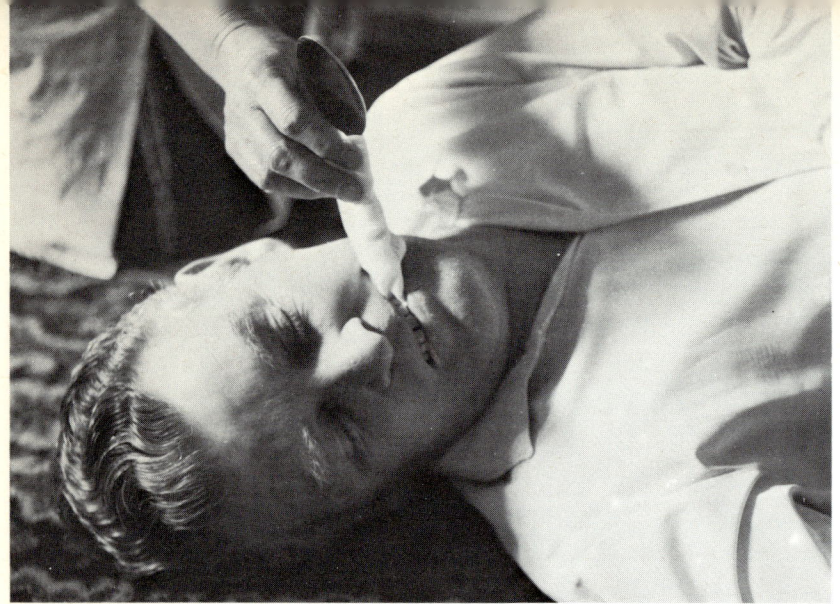

An improvised gag to protect the patient's tongue during fits.
A piece of wood is best, but a metal object can be padded with a
handkerchief. Note that it is introduced at the side of the mouth, far
back: front teeth are easily knocked out.

two of the patient's teeth are knocked out in the process! Most epileptic attacks are short, and followed by rapid recovery. The patient may not be as capable of looking after himself as he seems (he can sometimes walk and move, but does not know what he is doing); he could have another attack. He should at least be placed in the care of a friend, and not allowed to continue on his way alone, even if he seems determined to do so. All epileptic fits are not equally spectacular; some are very brief and quiet. Most people who are liable to what was once called 'the falling sickness' have in their wallet or handbag some tablets, or a hospital registration card, which will confirm the diagnosis.

Intoxication, whether due to *drugs* or *alcohol,* may be strongly indicated by the circumstances in which a casualty is found, but the diagnosis must not be made without caution. A man discovered unconscious outside a public house, and smelling strongly of alcohol, may have drunk no more than one small measure but may have fallen, fracturing his skull, as he left. Or he may have had a drink because he felt unwell, in an effort to stave off some illness which was the real cause of his collapse. The treatment of an individual who is unconscious through taking drugs or alcohol is discussed on pages 86–7 but, briefly, consists of placing him in a position in which he can breathe easily, watching his breathing and being ready to give artificial respiration if that stops.

OTHER CAUSES OF UNCONSCIOUSNESS

It may well be that, even after considering all three conditions you will have no indication that your patient is suffering from any of them. The probability then is that he is affected by some disease which could require expert investigation before it is certainly diagnosed. Perhaps he has had a stroke or is a diabetic? In such circumstances it is more important to make sure he does not asphyxiate, and to summon professional help, than to waste time pondering on the reason for his unconsciousness. If he is not breathing, or stops doing so while you are watching him, artificial respiration should be commenced, as described in the next chapter.

6
'He's not breathing' : the technique of artificial respiration

The facts that an individual is not moving, that he is not breathing, and that his heart cannot be felt beating must not be taken to imply that he is dead. At one time it was customary to begin any instructions about reviving the apparently dead by stating that only a doctor could pronounce life extinct. We now know that there are circumstances in which no one, even the most skilled physician, can trust his unaided senses but needs very sophisticated instruments before stating that a patient is certainly dead. The first-aider of course, may be confronted with injuries so gross that they are obviously fatal. In all other cases of recent apparent death, he must attempt to revive the victim, and should persist until a doctor's advice, or the development of certain changes, to be described later, suggest death has really occurred. The procedure is tiring and may seem hopeless, but while at work he may reflect upon the crest of the Royal Humane Society. That depicts a small cherub, blowing a fire which is only faintly smoking and the motto beneath is : '*Lateat scintillula forsan*' ('Perhaps a spark remains').

Having said resuscitation should be attempted, one must admit that there are many occasions when it is unlikely to succeed – and some where it is unnecessary! The extent of external wounds, and the circumstances in which a body is found, often indicate that even the most determined efforts at revival will fail. Do not

50

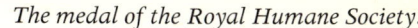
The medal of the Royal Humane Society.

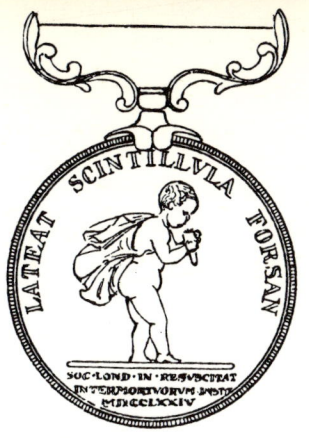

attach too much importance, though, to his temperature, for many instances have been reported of 'corpses' being revived even when they were stony-cold to the touch.

Do not give artificial respiration to a person who has collapsed because he is choking – at any rate, not until whatever is blocking the air passage has been removed. For instance, a man may suddenly and silently fall down while eating, because a large piece of meat has stuck in his throat: remove the obstruction and he may well breathe naturally. Do not give artificial respiration when the patient does not need it because he is breathing unaided. That may seem unnecessary advice but it is by no means rare to see a luckless individual (who has fainted, or had an epileptic fit) trying to breathe naturally while some well-meaning enthusiast squeezes his chest!

Artificial respiration is most likely to succeed when it is begun very shortly after natural breathing has ceased and it is not associated with any signs of gross external injury. These circumstances are most often found in three classes of patient – those who have been apparently electrocuted, those rescued from drowning, and those who have suffered a heart attack. The procedure to be followed in each case depends upon inflating the patient's lungs with air blown into them by the operator.

Methods advocated in the past involved compressing the patient's chest, to drive out any air remaining, allowing his lungs to fill again, and then forcing out the air once more. This cycle

51

was repeated for as long as necessary. Since this drives air in and out of any conscious person on whom it is rehearsed very effectively, you may well wonder why it has been superseded. The explanation lies in the difference between a normal chest and that of a patient dying of asphyxia. A healthy chest is springy and elastic. After air is expelled from it, the ribs and diaphragm rebound, sucking in more to replace it. Muscles deprived of oxygen have lost this resilience. The lungs do not fill again when the pressure on them is released and the air, which can be heard whistling in and out of a practice subject in such gratifying fashion, simply does not flow when it is really needed.

First-aiders are sometimes puzzled too, because the air blown into a patient by the 'mouth to mouth' technique now generally advocated, has been exhaled by his rescuer and has already been 'used'. While it is true that its oxygen content is slightly lower than that of fresh air, the difference is very small and insignificant. Inflating the patient's lungs with pure oxygen would be slightly better, and cylinders of gas are carried for this purpose on ambulances and fire-engines but the problem with which we are concerned now is that of keeping the patient alive until such equipment arrives.

THE TECHNIQUE

1 Work fast. Don't waste even half a minute by such measures as moving the patient on to a soft surface, or farther away from the water's edge.

2 Lay the patient on his back. This may not always be possible – if, for example, he has collapsed in a confined space, or is wedged inside a car. The first-aider must then weigh the necessity of starting respiration as soon as possible against the advantages of moving the patient into a position which will make resuscitation easier. Because it is quite possible to blow in some air with the casualty in almost any attitude, the general rule is: restore breathing first, and move him later.

3   Spend no more than two or three seconds checking that the air passages are clear. A finger is placed in the patient's mouth, and the back of his throat explored very swiftly to ensure it is not blocked by for example, weeds or pieces of food.

4   Kneel beside him, and tilt his head backwards. It is not enough to incline it slightly – push his forehead backwards with one hand, and lift his neck forwards with the other. Move his head as far back as it will easily go, until his nostrils are directed upwards.

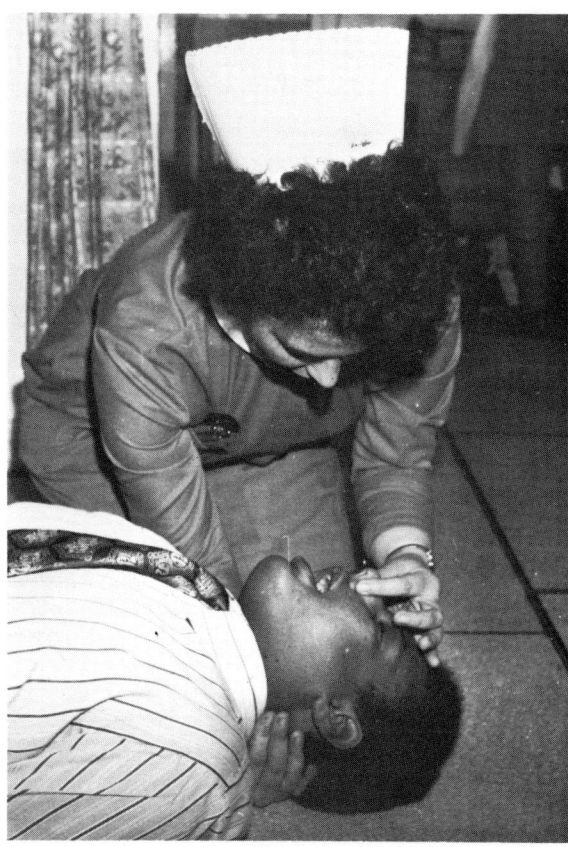

Preparing to administer mouth to mouth respiration. The patient's head must be tilted so far back that his nostrils are directed vertically upwards.

53

5 Now pinch the nostrils shut, using the forefinger and thumb of one hand: with the other, open the patient's mouth and cup your own lips around his, after first taking a deep breath.

6 Blow steadily, and you should see the patient's chest fill out. Raise your head, and take another breath. Then repeat the process of breathing into the casualty's mouth.

For the first minute, work very hard. Take deep breaths yourself, and pump them rapidly into the unconscious person, in an effort to give him some oxygen as quickly as possible. If you continue at such a rate you will soon feel dizzy, and may even faint, through disturbing the oxygen level of your own circulation. So after this rapid start, settle down to a steady, slower rate of about six or seven breaths per minute.

Sometimes air blown into the casualty's mouth travels, not down the windpipe into the lungs, but through the gullet into the stomach. When this occurs the abdomen swells instead of, or as well as, the chest. The first-aider should then pause long enough to press gently on the stomach with one hand, being ready with the other to turn the patient's head, and mop out his mouth, should the pressure cause vomiting.

If your efforts are successful, the casualty will begin taking short breaths himself, at irregular intervals. Adjust the rate of artificial respiration to his own breathing, and when that becomes regular, stop. It is important, though, to be prepared to start again if necessary. Unless your patient was unconscious for only a very short period, he will not open his eyes and speak, in the manner of film and television dramas! Whole days may elapse before that happens and he must be carefully watched meanwhile. There is a serious risk that his breathing may fail again during the first few hours.

One important point, often glossed over in books and lectures, remains for consideration. What do you do if the casualty does not begin breathing? The traditional answer is 'continue until he does, or until a doctor pronounces life extinct'. This advice, however, does not cover all possible situations. How long should a first-aider continue working on an individual who shows no sign of reviving when there are other casualties needing attention? How long should he continue when there is no doctor available, and none is likely to appear?

Obviously he must not give up lightly. Cases are on record of individuals being resuscitated only after two or three hours work by relays of volunteers. (Recovery after prolonged artificial respiration occurs more often for cases of apparent electrocution than after immersion in water, so a very sustained effort may be required when breathing has stopped following an electric shock.) If no doctor is available, artificial respiration should be continued for as long as possible – and perhaps just a little longer! The following signs, however, are an indication that no more can be done:

a the appearance of a dusky blue colouration, due to blood stagnating in the vessels just beneath the skin. It can be seen in the nape of the neck, the buttocks and the calf of the legs, if a casualty is lying on his back. This deep staining must be distinguished from a general congestion of the skin vessels, particularly those of the face, seen when a casualty is suffocating and in urgent need of resuscitation.

b a wide dilation of the pupils of the eye. Moderate dilation is often seen when respiration stops but, with effective ventilation of the lungs, the pupils should become smaller. A pupil which becomes more widely dilated, and does not close even when a bright light is shone into the eye at short range, is a bad sign.

7
Accidents at work

Industrial processes involve so many different materials and such a wide range of environments, that virtually every possible type of accident could be discussed under this heading. They may vary in degree from the trivial to the inevitably fatal but most have certain characteristics in common, which should reassure the first-aider. The majority of industrial accidents involve only one casualty and consequently involve no problem of priorities. Even if more than one person is injured, the first-aider will usually have plenty of help. He is unlikely to find himself short of the bandages, splints and dressings which are often lacking in other situations and, paradoxically, he will never need them less, since professional assistance will usually be forthcoming, often within a few minutes.

This chapter deals with three very grave situations and two which are more common but less serious – though still distressing enough to the unfortunate casualty.

APPARENT ELECTROCUTION OR ASPHYXIATION

Both of these are desperate emergencies. No matter how elaborate the works' medical facilities are, they may be useless unless the first person who realises what has happened takes the appropriate action. It is essentially the same in both cases: get the casualty to safety and get him breathing. Reduce the risk and restore respiration!

Rescuing someone who has had an electric shock is a much less dangerous manoeuvre than is commonly supposed. Only seldom is he 'held on' to the electrical circuit, and contact will usually be broken when he falls. When a person is still connected to the current source, any would-be rescuer who touches him may receive a shock – but the casualty's body is interposed and constitutes a resistance which reduces the effective voltage. If a first-aider is wearing dry clothes, and envelops his hands in dry insulating material (for instance, the sleeves of his reversed jacket) he is unlikely to harm himself when knocking an unconscious patient from a 200-400 volt source. A much greater risk is posed by conductors carrying very high voltages, such as those flowing through the wires on grid supply pylons. It may be impossible to move a casualty from them until they have been made safe, even though the switching-off operation costs time.

Retrieving a man who has collapsed in the gases filling a tank or sewer is very different. The dangers are not so evident, but much greater. Instances of one electrical fatality being immediately followed by another are rare but every year many rescuers succumb while trying to pull a person out of a gas-filled space. Examples of three and even four successive deaths are not unusual. Each case must be considered individually and with regard to the character of the fumes involved. Remember though, that it is impossible to hold one's breath and move an inert body at the same time, and that such devices as a handkerchief tied over the nose and mouth are, in most cases, literally worse than useless. Even several layers of cloth, whether dry or moist, have no effect on most poisonous gases and vapours and merely encumber the wearer. Rescues from poisonous gases must be concerted, and well planned. The individual who attempts one on his own would usually render more valuable service by summoning help, trying to create a ventilation draught and finding some rope.

Once the casualty is in safe surroundings, begin artificial respiration. The standard mouth-to-mouth method is usually advocated but some people think that methods which entail compressing the chest and lifting (explained on pages 51–2) are better in apparent electrocution since, if the heart has stopped, such movements may stimulate it to beat again. Whichever method is practised, it should be used promptly, maintained without interruption and continued for as long as possible. An individual who appears to be dead after an electric shock may respond to resuscitation efforts only after half an hour or longer. Such delayed recoveries are rare after apparent drowning.

MACHINE ACCIDENTS

These may confront the first-aider with a very testing situation. Some are trivial as, for instance, the superficial lacerations inflicted by a small metal fragment spinning from a lathe. Others involve the crushing of several fingers or a whole hand, and leave the casualty still trapped in the mechanism. The hands and upper limbs, of course, suffer much more often than the legs and feet. Here are a few guiding rules:

a   If the casualty is trapped when the machine stops, send for help and do not be tempted to try to pull him free. Above all, remember that reversing a machine is almost always wrong, because the tissues will be further damaged by a second passage under its rollers or cogs.

b   A casualty in a machine may be frightened and suffering from nervous shock but, during the period immediately after injury, is not often in pain, or bleeding dangerously. So proceed very deliberately. It may be necessary to prise open or disassemble the mechanism, and, while this is being done, prepare a stretcher, call an ambulance, and reassure the patient.

c   Plenty of loose fluffy gauze, with a firm bandage over it, is the ideal dressing.

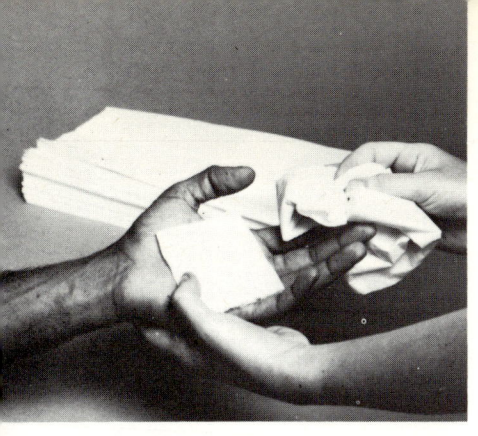 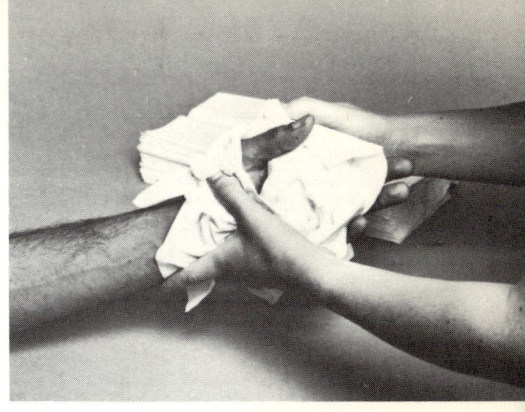

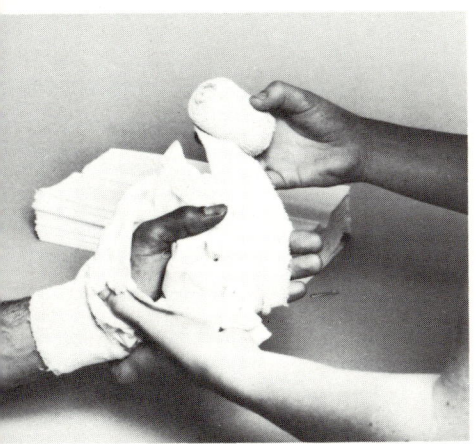 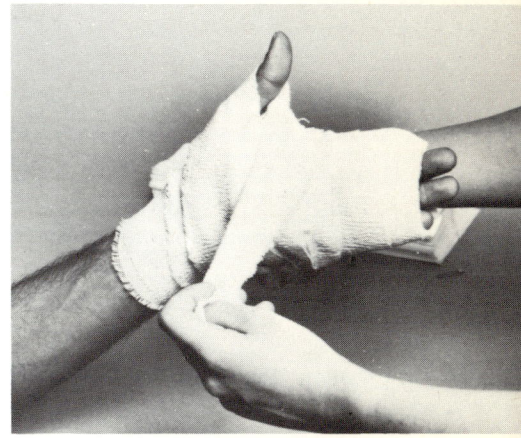

Bandaging a damaged hand. The cleanest available dressing is applied to any wound, then bulky pieces of soft compressible material are applied to the back, front and sides of the hand. Fluffed out gauze is ideal, but crumpled paper towels are used here. They are held in place by a bandage which exerts uniform pressure and should impart a final appearance reminiscent of a boxing glove, perhaps a little tighter than that shown here.

d An injured man can be allowed to smoke. He may need an anaesthetic later, so give him nothing by mouth.

e Pieces of skin and other tissues which have separated, should be placed in the cleanest possible dry container and taken with the patient to hospital. Every now and again some of these can be utilised to repair the damage.

A person may on occasion fall from even a second storey and escape serious harm. Alternatively, a stumble over a kerbstone can cause an open fracture at the ankle. The injuries described here are those which typically follow a drop of twenty or thirty feet or more on to a hard surface. The first-aider is faced with a huddled figure, almost certainly seriously hurt, and may be at a loss to know how to begin. It is essential that he should know what injuries to expect and the priority with which they should be treated:

a   If the patient is unconscious, examine his head. If there is no obvious bump or bleeding at the back and top of the skull he is probably either concussed, or has a fracture through the base of the skull. Both conditions can occur without the head actually hitting the ground, as a result of the shock transmitted along the spine.

b   Feel along the lower limbs, starting at one ankle, working upwards to the hip, and then down the opposite leg. Be on the look out for swelling and deformity round the knee or ankle or in the thigh. These are common sites for 'deceleration fractures'. Move each hip cautiously. (Tenderness, or feeling a difference between the bony contours of the two hips, would suggest a fracture or dislocation.) Then, again gently, squeeze the crests of the hip bones together, noting whether the patient stirs or winces as you do so. If he does, this might indicate a pelvic fracture.

c   Without moving the casualty, pass a hand up and down his back, to find out whether he has any gross damage to the spine: if he can co-operate, confirm that his legs are not paralysed and then run your hands over the chest and abdomen looking for any tenderness which might suggest rib fractures or internal injuries.

When the first diagnostic check is completed, apply bandages (and if they are available, splints) as appropriate. The legs can be splinted by tying them together, and one or two broad bandages (or scarves) round the hips will help to immobilise a broken pelvis. Raise the legs and lower the head, to combat shock. If time permits, feel the patient's upper limbs, and check the lower ones again – fractures of the heel bones and wrist should be sought.

A WRENCHED BACK

This is a very common, and often dramatic, event. A man who is lifting a heavy load, or who has to turn suddenly, cries out in pain and is unable to straighten up. His distress is so evident that his colleagues are afraid to touch him. The condition often occurs in some difficult situation – so when the first-aider arrives, the biggest problem confronting him may be how to get the patient down from a height, or up a steep flight of steps.

Just what causes such sudden severe pain is still disputed even by orthopaedic specialists – perhaps a ligament is strained, a muscle torn, or part of the lining of a joint is nipped. The condition always subsides with rest, and is never followed by any permanent disability. Once this is realised, the emergency seems much less formidable.

a Find out what has happened from the patient, and any witnesses. Only if they describe a heavy fall, or a hard blow, must the case be regarded as a possible spinal fracture, and handled accordingly.

b If there has been no such injury and the individual has indeed hurt himself only by some movement he made, reassure him and feel his back carefully. You will learn nothing but, while doing this, talk to him and gain his confidence. Defuse the situation as much as possible – stretchers and special carrying harnesses are not necessary. Instead reassure the patient and encourage him to make his own way, as slowly as he likes and with the help of one or two supporters, to any room in which there is a comfortable couch. The heat of a water-bottle, and a couple of Paracetamol tablets, will then work wonders.

Statistics show that this is an injury to the foot – particularly the big toe – from a falling weight and that is the reason why everyone handling heavy loads should wear boots with reinforced toecaps. In its commonest form, this accident is painful and likely to cause lengthy incapacity, but is not otherwise serious.

When the patient's shoes have been removed, there may be little visible abnormality. More often though, the nail is discoloured by bleeding underneath it. The blood may ooze from

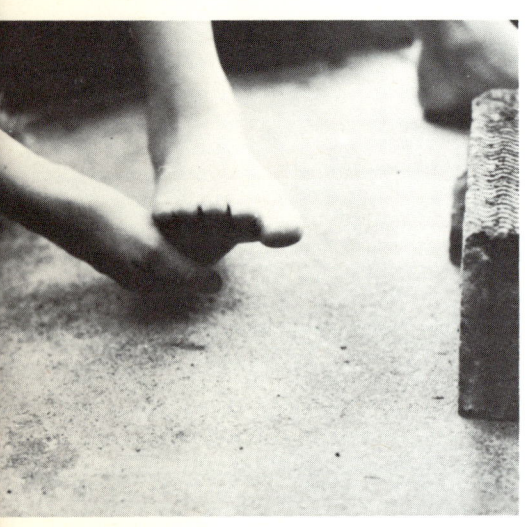
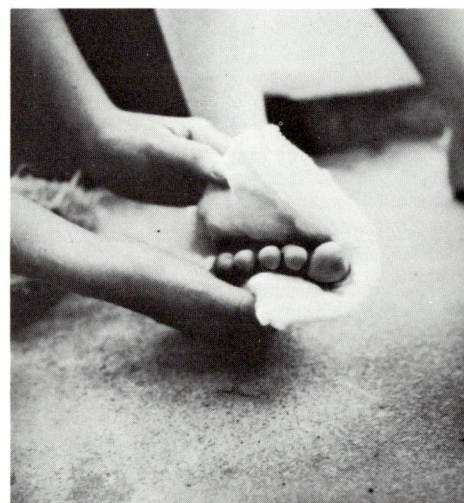
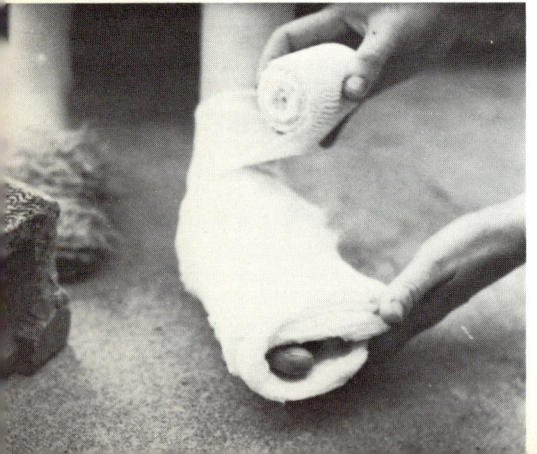
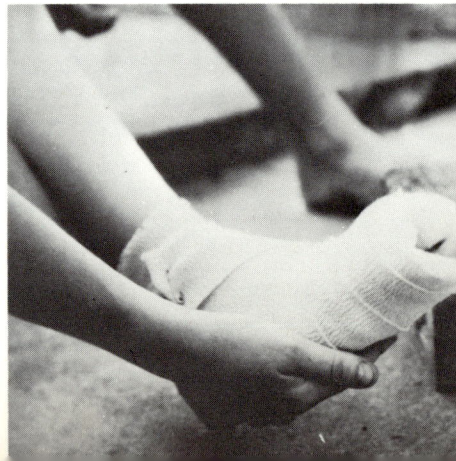

beneath the edges of the nail, and sometimes the whole nail is loose. Bandaging such a toe is difficult and painful – leave the nail undisturbed, place a loose mass of cotton-wool or gauze round all the toes and apply a bandage over this. Lotions, cold compresses and the like should be avoided if there is any evidence of bleeding, because that indicates an open wound which may communicate with a crack in the toe bone. It is, in fact, an open fracture in miniature, and bathing it could introduce infection.

Finally, it is worth noting that injuries to fingers produced by a misdirected hammer blow (so-called 'handyman's thumb'), are almost identical to those caused to the toes by falling objects and, therefore, are treated in the same way.

An injured foot should be surrounded by a loose mass of cotton-wool or gauze which is held in place by a bandage. A more uniform pressure will be exerted by a bandage a little tighter than that demonstrated here.

8
Domestic disasters

'Safe as houses' is not really a very accurate metaphor. Every day hundreds of people sustain injuries, and sometimes dangerous injuries, inside their own homes. Some houses, because their occupants have eliminated such things as loose carpets in dark corners and worn electric leads, are safer than others. In any house two rooms are likely to be more hazardous than the rest – the kitchen and the bathroom. The high incidence of kitchen accidents is easily understood, for that is where the sharp cutlery, the hot stove and perhaps the gas point are located; the bathroom is dangerous because of such risks as slippery surfaces, boiling water, radiators, electric supply points and poisonous lotions or disinfectants.

This chapter is concerned with two types of accident in particular – falls, and burns or scalds. It is also convenient to consider here some miscellaneous conditions which occur from time to time in even the 'best regulated households', such as bleeding from the nose or from varicose veins.

FALLS AT HOME

There are two very common fractures – one at the wrist, the other near the hip joint – which occur more frequently in women during the second half of life than in any other group in the population. For that reason, they are encountered more often indoors than out though occasionally, of course, they are seen in other individuals and other environments. Both injuries have one thing in common – only slight violence may be needed to cause them, particularly in elderly subjects. For that reason and because there is not always a gross deformity, they may not be recognised at first.

COLLES' FRACTURE

This is named after the Irish surgeon, Abraham Colles, who first described it. The two bones which comprise the forearm are broken at their lower ends, just above the wrist joint, as a result of a fall on the outstretched hand. Sometimes the fracture can be diagnosed at a glance, from the manner in which the hand is displaced, the so called 'dinner-fork' deformity. (See illustration.)

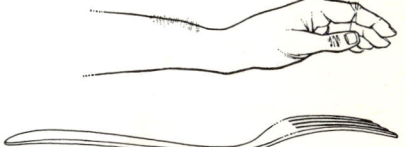

The 'dinner-fork' deformity of Colles' fracture.

If the bone fragments have not moved much, and have been driven together (impacted) the wrist, though painful and slightly swollen, may look almost normal.

It is easy then to dismiss the condition as a sprain (that is, as a tear of the ligaments which fasten the hand bones to the arm). In fact, sprains at the wrist joint are very rare, and Colles' fractures very common. So anyone with a painful wrist, following even a light fall, should be treated for a fracture even if there is no obvious damage.

Because the bone ends are jammed together, there is no tendency for the wrist to wobble about in an abnormal manner or for the forearm to bend at an unnatural level; so splinting is not necessary. A firm bandage may relieve some of the discomfort and the arm should be placed in a sling. The patient should then be seen by a doctor.

Though children or young adults can sustain a fracture of the upper end of the femur, this part of their skeleton is so strong that they seldom do. In women over the age of about sixty, however, the neck of the thigh bone becomes more brittle and will sometimes snap if the individual merely stumbles on a loose rug, or falls out of bed.

As with a Colles' fracture, the diagnosis may be obvious or difficult. Typically there is considerable pain, a complete inability to walk, and a characteristic deformity – the foot turns outwards and the patient cannot rotate it back into a normal position. Sometimes though, she may be unaware of having hurt herself and may be able to walk with only a slight limp and very

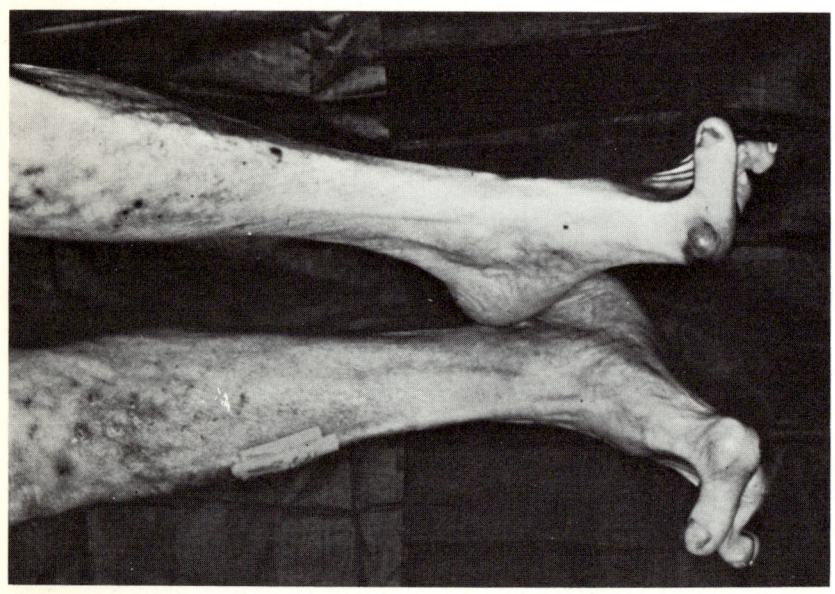

It is a characteristic deformity of a broken hip that the foot turns outward and the patient is unable to rotate it back to a normal position.

little pain. This state of affairs can be dangerous if unrecognised and neglected, for the bone fragments which have been impacted (that is, driven into each other), may separate days or weeks later, producing a sudden, very gross, and disabling deformity.

If a 'broken hip bone' is suspected, do not let the casualty even attempt to walk. Fasten the ankles together (thereby restoring the

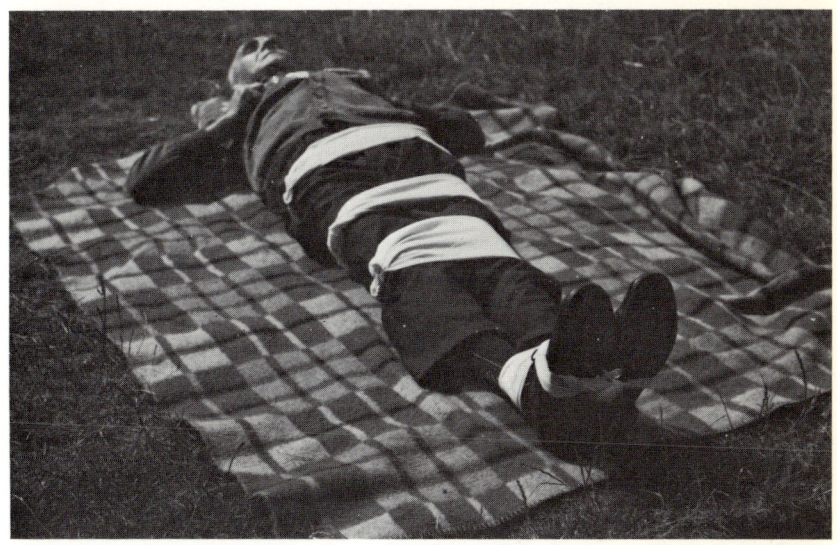

If a broken hip is suspected the feet should be bandaged
together in normal alignment and if possible
additional bandages tied around the hips, knees and thighs.

ordinary alignment of the foot, if that was rotated) and apply additional bandages round the hips, knees and thighs. Carry the patient carefully, and arrange for removal to hospital on a stretcher rather than, for example, sitting in a car.

These two common injuries are treated, in other words, along the basic guide lines laid down in chapter 3. That is to say, once the possibility of a fracture is appreciated, the limb is immobilised before the patient is moved. It is customary to add 'and he or she is treated for shock' but, in fact, these two particular fractures are so often the result of relatively little violence that any considerable degree of shock is unusual. A casualty, particularly at home, is nevertheless likely to be given the traditional cup of hot, sweet tea and it is worth repeating that no food or drink should be given to anybody who is going to hospital, and who might need an anaesthetic during the next four hours.

BURNS AND SCALDS

The very first thing to do immediately you, or anyone else, has been burnt or scalded, is to plunge the injured part into cold water: if the area – say the chest or thigh – cannot be placed under a tap, or in a wash basin, throw a container of cold water over it, take off any clothing which can easily be removed, and cover the affected part with towels, dishcloths or handkerchiefs which are wringing wet.

A burn or scald should be treated by immediate immersion in cold water, if that is available. Otherwise wet towels, cloths or handkerchiefs should be used to cover the injury.

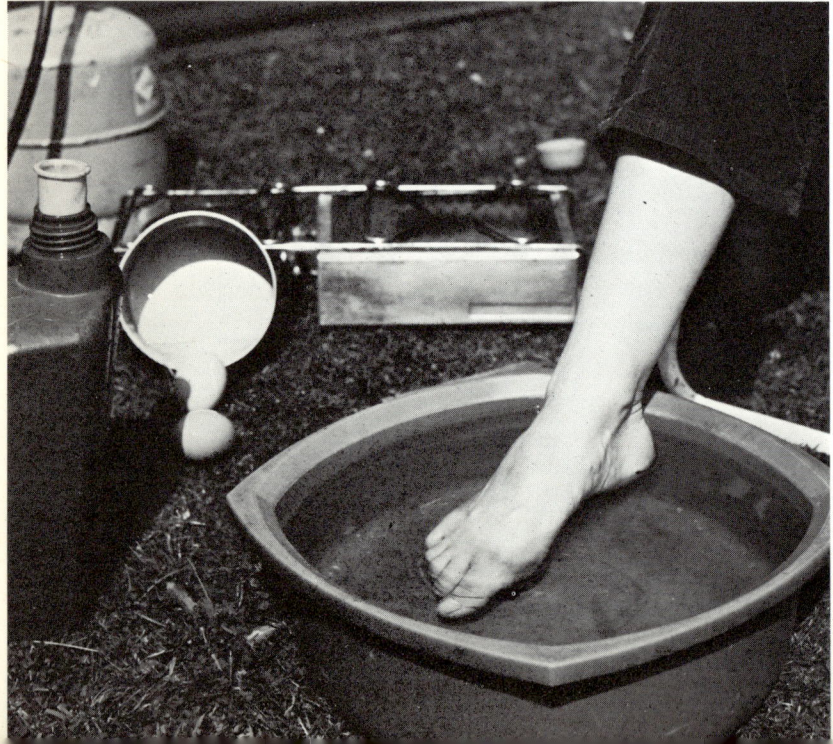

The object of this procedure is to cool the region and cut short the effects of heat. After burning, the tissues of the body, once raised above their normal temperature, may go on 'cooking' for several minutes, causing the damage to increase. So cooling may be beneficial even when as long as five or even ten minutes has elapsed, especially if the temperatures reached were very high, or clothing is retaining the heat.

There is no essential difference between a burn (which is due to dry heat) and a scald (which is due to moist heat – either from hot liquids, or the vapour given off from them). In practice, the very great majority of scalds are due to water, which cannot under ordinary atmospheric conditions be heated above 100°C. (212°F). So scalds, in general, are less severe than burns (due to dry heat, from sources of very variable, and often very high, temperature). Both are treated in the same way.

Let us suppose that the damaged tissues have been effectively cooled by immersion in cold water – or that if, unfortunately, cold water was not immediately available, some was subsequently poured over them. What is to be done next? That will depend upon the depth and extent of the injury and we can define three broad classes:

a *The common trivial burn* due, for example, to momentary contact with a cigarette end or an electric iron. This will heal quickly and without any special treatment. The initial pain controlled by a dressing which keeps the air away – petroleum jelly or cold cream serves very well. If the heat is intense, or acts for more than a fraction of a second, a blister may form. This should be kept intact for as long as possible, since it protects the raw tissues beneath and reduces the risk of infection. If the burn is deep – as shown by some browning or blackening of the tissues – a doctor should see it, even if the area is very small, since infection and a long delay in healing may ensue.

b *A burn involving a wider area.* Commonly such burns vary in depth from one part to another – in places the skin will be red and tender but unbroken; at others, blistered, or frankly charred. The ointments and creams used for lesser burns should not be used – the patient needs treatment by a doctor, and such preparations interfere with his assessment of the damage and with surgical cleansing if that is necessary. Instead apply compresses of gauze, handkerchiefs, face flannels or other clean materials, soaked in cold or tepid water. If the patient has to move about or be moved, fasten over these plenty of fluffed out cotton-wool and bandages, using no more pressure than is necessary to keep the compresses in position. A scorched face or burnt chest can be covered with a sheet or towel, again soaked in water, but with holes cut to allow the casualty to breathe and see.

c *Deep burns of a small area.* These are most often seen on the hands, and are the result of more prolonged contact with a very hot surface or with a source of electric current. They are characterised by charring of the skin, and by the development within a few days of an ulcer (that is, a hole in the skin). Because, as indicated above, they may prove slow to heal, such burns should be seen by a doctor as soon as conveniently possible. Meanwhile they should be cooled in water, and then covered with the cleanest available dressing.

NOSE BLEEDS

Bleeding from the nose is often due to a blow, sometimes (in children) to a mild infection or inflammation, for example, aggravated by picking; occasionally to other causes – for example, raised blood pressure. The bleeding in the majority of cases ceases quickly and spontaneously and this explains why any of a wide variety of treatments seems effective. A more profuse loss, which shows no sign of stopping, is alarming but should be dealt with as follows.

Make the patient sit down. (Walking about not only pumps out blood more rapidly – it causes more mess!) Give him a cork, pencil,

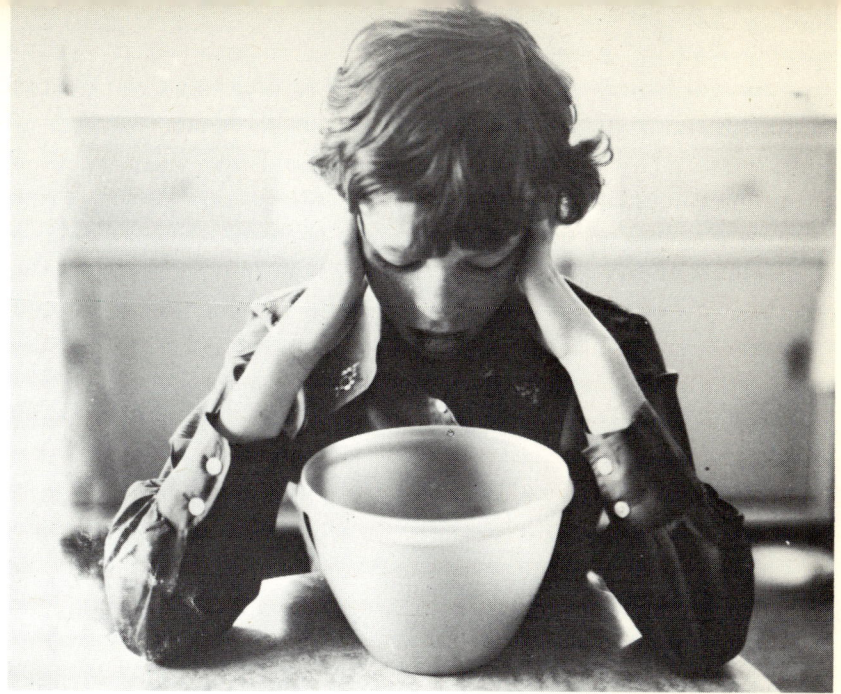

*To stop a nosebleed the patient should support his head over a basin or
bucket and hold a small object, a cork in this case, between his teeth.*

indiarubber or similar object to hold between his teeth (this is
said to contract some of the muscles in the nose and throat, and to
facilitate clot formation in the open vessels). Place a basin or
bucket in front of him, and let him support over it his head,
resting on his hands. Blood and saliva may continue draining into
the receptacle for five or ten minutes but, if the patient does not
keep taking out the object between his teeth, talking, or raising
his head, the bleeding almost invariably ceases within this
period.

BLEEDING FROM A VARICOSE VEIN

During the second half of life and sometimes earlier, grossly
dilated veins may appear on the inner side of the thighs, or on the
calfs of the legs. The causes and treatment of these 'varicose
veins' need not concern us here but it is important to know that

the veins sometimes give rise to bleeding which is always very alarming and, if not properly treated, could be fatal.

The skin over them is often thin, poorly nourished and sometimes very friable and scaly ('varicose eczema'). If this gives way, profuse bleeding can follow – made the more spectacular if the patient runs about in a terrified effort to stop it. Actually, the pressure in these veins is quite low, and the haemorrhage very easy to control. It suffices simply to make the patient lie down and raise his foot up in the air – perhaps resting it on a stool, or the seat of a chair. A pad and bandage will take care of any continued oozing.

The bleeding can be stopped, irrespective of the patient's position, and while someone else is looking for a bandage, by placing two thumbs on the vein itself. One is applied just below the ulcerated area which is bleeding (that is, between the ulcer and the ankle) and the other just above it. When these veins bleed, they do so from both ends, unlike healthy ones which have 'valves' along their length.

9
Injuries at play

The misadventures that befall us during our recreation are almost as varied as those which happen at work – but, if injuries from falling objects, lacerations from sharp edges, and falls from a height, are frequent hazards of industry, they are relatively rare at play. Instead we are likely to damage our limbs through our own exertions, to suffer from unexpected changes in climate and – at the end of the scale – from the unwelcome attention of irritating animals. This chapter deals with the commonest of these miscellaneous troubles.

FOOTBALL INJURIES

Apart from bruises, sprains, and the occasional case of mild concussion, footballers most often need medical attention for fractures of the collar bone and, much less often, for those in the shin or near the ankle. These have been described in chapter 3 but there is one injury which is particularly associated with a football field – a torn cartilage in the knee.

There are two cartilages in each knee – crescent-shaped pieces of (as their names implies) gristle, interposed between the ends of the thigh and the shin bones. If these bones are twisted against each other (characterically, by a player changing direction suddenly, by turning his body whilst his foot is still firmly on the ground) one or other of the cartilages may split, causing a sickening pain and instant disability. The diagnosis can often be made from the touchline for the man drops to the ground, without having been heavily tackled, and lies there holding his knee. Closer examination shows the joint is bent, but cannot be bent further, or straightened, without causing severe pain.

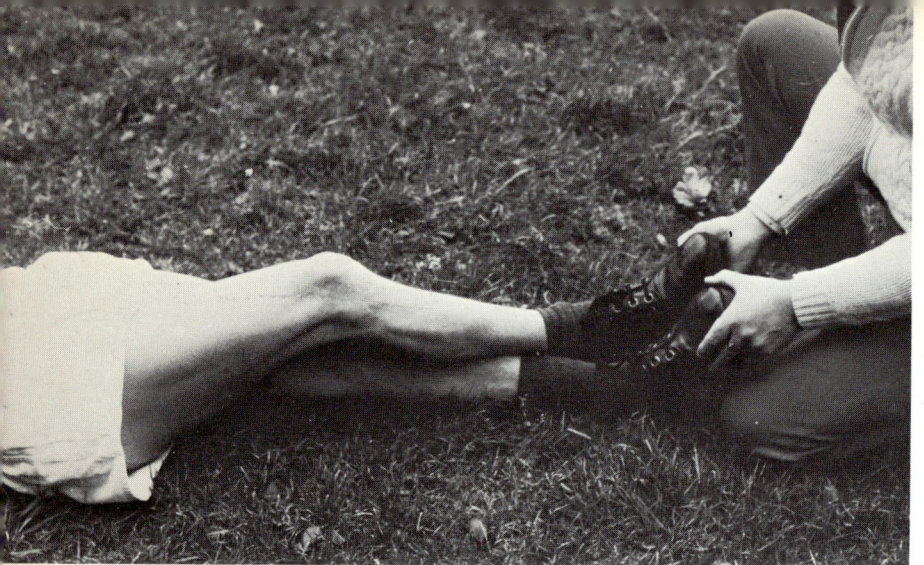

Immobilising a suspected cartilage injury. If the legs are crossed and then tied together at the knees and ankles the casualty can be carried more comfortably.

The condition requires skilled attention, and even moving the patient can be difficult if the joint is very painful. Enveloping his knee in a thick jacket of cotton-wool, under a firm crepe bandage, will afford some relief and if he remains unable to walk, he can be carried on a stretcher with the injured knee, still bent, crossed over the opposite one.

HEAT STROKE

An inhabitant of the British Isles very rarely develops heat stroke at home. On holiday abroad he may suffer from it while undertaking unusual exertions in a hot climate, particularly if the air is humid and still. Under such conditions the body's temperature-regulating mechanism breaks down, because perspiration does not evaporate.

Heat stroke has a sudden onset – the victim is irritable, complains of headache and fatigue, and then becomes confused, or even unconscious. His condition may well become critical unless his skin, which is very hot and dry to the touch, is cooled as rapidly as possible. All his clothes must be removed, and a routine of sponging with cold water, and of fanning the victim (mechanically, or by hand) continued until he improves.

COLD EXHAUSTION

The reverse condition – cold exhaustion – every year claims several victims who had no idea they were at risk from it. These are often young people, caught in the open by deteriorating weather for which they were unprepared. Its onset is more insidious than the effects of a raised temperature and the signs may be mistaken for simply the manifestations of fatigue – irritability, slowness, and a difficulty in making decisions. This mental failure, unfortunately, may prevent the sufferer from taking the steps essential for his own safety – such as changing his route for a shorter one or, if no such route exists, from looking for what shelter he can find while he is still strong enough to do so.

Dealing with a potential case of cold exhaustion is a subject for books on survival techniques, rather than first aid but, in general, it is better to stop, revive the casualty, and make what one can of prevailing conditions, rather than to stagger on and risk a dangerous collapse. Confronted on a rescue mission by a developed case, the first-aider will find the patient very cold, dazed, or unconscious, and with a slow heart and breathing rate. Very obviously he must be warmed but not too rapidly. Often the most practical and sensible step is to enclose the casualty in a sleeping-bag and put one of the rescue party in beside him, after the outer clothing of both individuals has been removed. As soon as possible, the patient should be put to bed in a warm room and given plenty of hot drinks when he is able to swallow. Do not try to warm him quickly by using electric blankets or very warm baths or open fires at short range – because, since the patient's skin is cold, and little blood is flowing through it, such methods are less effective in raising his internal temperature than one might expect and they are very likely to burn him.

True frostbite is a consequence of very low temperatures maintained for a long time and in the British Isles this is distinctly unusual. In our normally temperate climate the victims are more often vagrants, fugitives and the mentally enfeebled, rather than genuine travellers or tourists.

The parts of the body affected are those which always first 'feel the cold' that is, the fingers and toes, the nose and ears. Sustained chilling of these extremities causes a pallor and numbness which

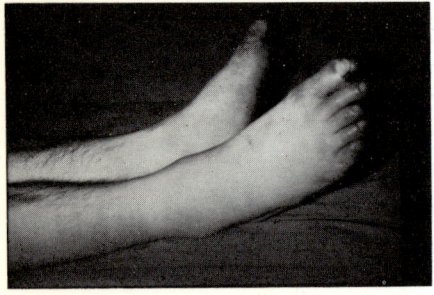

Frostbite. Pallor or numbness in the affected area may deteriorate to a blue or black discolouration.

may progress to a blue and black discolouration and then, actual separation of the damaged tissues. Treatment depends on restoring the circulation but not by massaging or applying direct heat (which could aggravate the condition). Instead, warm the patient as a whole and, if necessary, the fingers or toes themselves, by tucking them inside your own jacket.

FOREIGN BODIES IN THE EYE

The great majority of tiny objects which enter the eye (smuts from a fire, tiny insects and the like) come to rest under the lower lid: most of the rest are to be found under the upper one.
They should be removed as follows:
1   Sit the patient in a good light but not facing one which is so strong as to irritate his eye.

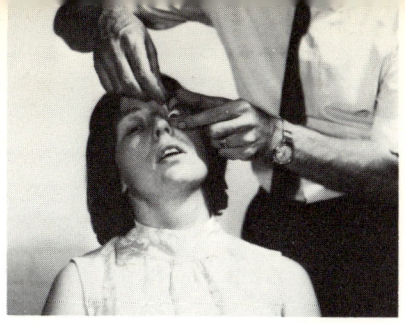

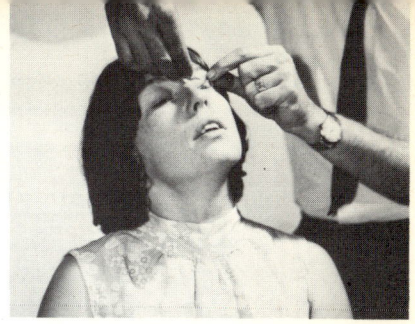

Using a wisp of cotton wool to remove a foreign body from the eye.

How to evert the upper eyelid. Of course, this must be done with very great care.

2   Stand behind him, tilt his head towards you, and pull down his lower lid.

3   If you can see the foreign body resting inside it, remove it with a wisp of soft material. The corner of a handkerchief is generally used but a small wisp of cotton-wool, smeared with castor-oil or liquid paraffin, is better.

4   If the offending object is not there, tell the patient to close his eye and look down. Place a matchstick along the upper edge of the upper lid and turn the lid 'inside out' by grasping the lashes gently, and rolling the eyelid upwards against the matchstick. The foreign body will now often be seen lying in the centre of the lid.

Foreign bodies which are travelling fast, for example grains of blown sand or small particles from grindstones used without protective clothing, may embed themselves on the front of the eye. They are not then easily recognised but if seen, they may be dislodged by a very light touch. There can be no question of using anything except a wisp of oiled cotton-wool for this, and only one or two attempts are permissible. By persevering longer, you may aggravate the situation by scratching the very delicate tissue covering of the eye, so instil a drop of castor-oil or liquid paraffin and apply a pad and bandage until a doctor is available.

His advice must be sought, also, if any irritation continues after a foreign body has been removed and, of course, if there is any suggestion that the surface of the eye has been penetrated by glass splinters or other sharp objects.

INSECT STINGS

In the past it was said that bee or wasp stings were best dabbed with an acid or an alkali and the first-aider's chief difficulty lay in trying to remember which was the appropriate remedy. In fact, neither made much difference and the same is true, unfortunately, even of modern anti-histamine creams. Though some authorities claim that such creams help if used within one or two minutes, the irritant substance has been injected under the skin and remedies rubbed on the surface of the body do not neutralise its effect. Bathing, cold compresses and eau-de-cologne will minimise the swelling if used at once and later, calamine lotion or sunburn preparations will reduce the itching.

SNAKE BITES

Only one venomous snake is native to the British Isles – the adder: it is not very poisonous. Its bite causes pain, followed by considerable swelling and some bruising. Serious upsets such as vomiting, abdominal pain and collapse may follow but they are distinctly unusual and deaths are almost unknown. It is important to realise this and to know that these effects wear off spontaneously within twenty-four or forty-eight hours, because the principal dangers come, not from the bite itself, but from the wrong kind of treatment. The essential points to remember are negative ones – don't panic; don't apply a tourniquet; don't above all, attempt such heroic measures as incising, cauterising or sucking the wound. Instead, reassure the casualty in emphatic terms: kill and keep the snake if you can. Rest the bitten part, if it is on a limb, by immobilising it as much as if there were a fracture. Ideally, the patient should then rest and be carried to a doctor; more often, he will have to proceed under his own power, without undue exertion or haste.

10
The car crash

In an ideal existence a first-aider's first cases would be individuals with cut fingers, or who were feeling faint and he would progress by way of minor sprains to simple fractures, and so on. Unfortunately, it is one of the facts of life that his earliest test is very likely to be a major road accident, in which he has to deal simultaneously with several seriously injured people. In such circumstances, confronted by more than one casualty, a great deal of broken glass, and sometimes a fair amount of blood, it is important to remember that the possible injuries – cuts, fractures, concussion – are basically those we have already discussed, and that the principles for dealing with them are the same, whatever the scene in which they are encountered. The same order of procedure holds good:

1   Make sure no further injuries are likely to be produced. Check that nobody is likely to be hit by other vehicles and that those which are damaged are not about to burst into flames.
2   Attend to any casualty who is not breathing, and do what you can to restore respiration.
3   Look for any profuse bleeding and stop it.

These general rules may have to be modified in some circumstances, for the assessment of the overall situation can be the most difficult part of roadside first aid. When a crash has blocked the road just beyond a blind corner, there is no doubt that, even if there are several badly hurt people trapped, the most urgent and sensible step towards helping them is to ensure that, another vehicle does not crash. It may be possible to detail someone to wave down oncoming drivers, or warn them by laying out in the road such objects as tools or clothing. (By night, a row of four hub-caps provides an audible, as well as visible, signal). Pause for a few seconds to consider, too, whether you yourself are in danger of being knocked down and becoming a casualty – policemen and ambulance crews are supplied with 'high visibility' waistcoats but the best alternative is to work in a light-coloured shirt or dress. This may mean taking off a dark coat; at night or in poor weather at least tie a white scarf, or several handkerchiefs, or a triangular bandage round your neck or waist. Any leakage of petrol from a crashed vehicle particularly suggests a fire hazard but in any case, it is a sensible precaution to isolate the battery by unscrewing its terminals (the earth one first, to eliminate sparking!).

Individuals who have extricated themselves unaided have a lesser claim upon your attention than those who are still inside a car. Check that the latter are not trapped, bleeding or in any respiratory difficulty. If, however, they are not in any danger from fire, do not be in too great a hurry to pull them out. A serious injury may be aggravated by careless handling; even someone who is not badly hurt may be better off inside a car than lying on a cold wet surface. One final point about the assessment of casualties – make sure you have indeed seen all of them. Under conditions of bad visibility, motor cyclists who have been thrown over a hedge, or injured people who have staggered a few yards before collapsing, have often been overlooked.

CHARACTERISTIC INJURIES

As we have already said, the injuries encountered on the highway are those seen elsewhere, so they include such conditions as concussion, a broken shin-bone or a heart attack. Certain injuries are particularly common and we shall consider these in some detail.

Cuts and skin wounds are most often seen on the head and hands, from contact with the windscreen. No special treatment is indicated but they are often multiple and deep. Even a little blood smeared over the face is frightening, and it is reassuring to remember that most of such wounds look worse than they really are. (Permanent disfigurement after road accidents is surprisingly rare – but that is not a good reason for neglecting one's safety belt!)

Fractures are likely to involve the ribs and the lower limbs, particularly the knee and thigh. The broken ribs are due to the chest striking the sides of the car or, in the case of the driver, the steering-wheel. Their effects vary from no more than a sharp pain in the side, which is worse on breathing, and on pressure over the damaged area, to a very extensive distortion of the chest. This 'stove-in' deformity only occurs if many ribs have been broken and is dangerous because, by interfering with the expansion of the lungs, it causes shock and a very serious collapse. Treatment in either case should be confined to reassuring the patient (anxiety, and uncontrolled panting increases his difficulties) and relieving the pain. In general, he will be more comfortable lying on the injured side, because the broken ribs then move less and the intact side of his chest can function to the best advantage. Sometimes the patient feels better if left in the car where he can steady his arms and part of his chest against the wheel. Putting tight bandages or adhesive strapping round him could aggravate the damage, so do not use them without a doctor's advice. If the patient feels better when holding his side, the effect of a scarf or broad bandage, over his clothes can be tried.

The most typical of all automobile fractures are those across the knee cap, and those in which the upper end of the thigh bone breaks against the pelvis. Both are due to the person shooting violently forwards, so that his knee strikes the dashboard or some projection below it. Each is easily recognised by the pain and because the patient is quite unable to walk or stand. There is usually a deformity but it may be slight, or obscured by swelling. When such fractures are suspected, they are dealt with by tying the limbs together, so that one splints the other (see chapter 3).

While this seldom presents much difficulty, it is not unusual for a fracture at the upper end of the thigh to be associated with damage to the hip joint. In that case the leg, twisted up or sideways, may be too painful to straighten and the first-aider must immobilise it as best he can – after, for instance, placing a pillow or rolled-up coat under both knees.

Injuries to the upper part of the spine – the neck bones – are also frequent. Fortunately, the most common, a sprain of the neck, is painful rather than at all dangerous. It usually happens when the patient is sitting in a stationary car and another vehicle runs into it from behind. His head shoots violently forwards, then backwards: several hours later, rather than immediately afterwards, his neck becomes so stiff that any movement is excruciating. He must be examined in hospital, but a deep collar can be improvised out of, for example, a folded newspaper, to help him to get there.

A rarer, and much more serious situation is that in which the neck has been exposed to so much violence that its bones have become displaced on each other. This usually happens when the patient has been thrown against the roof or through the windscreen, often with so much force that he has lost consciousness. The particular danger of such injuries is that the spinal cord may have been damaged, and he may suffer still more harm from any further movement of the neck. So, if an occupant of a crashed car, particularly on a front seat, stays huddled up and motionless, be in no hurry to pull him out. Loosen his clothing to help his breathing and, if he needs artificial respiration, consider administering this by getting in beside him, tilting his head as little as possible, and having someone else support it. Emergency vehicles carry special splints to immobilise the neck in such cases but, if none is available, the collar described above, or a short plank, fastened to the patient's back by bandages round the chest and forehead, may have to serve instead.

Bad weather may necessitate keeping casualties inside a car. It is also often the best place for those only slightly hurt or those who, because of injuries to the jaws and face, are most comfortable in a sitting position. Remember that when shock threatens, the patient should be laid down, with his legs raised. A satisfactory arrangement is to place him beside the car (on seats taken from it) and at right angles to it: his legs can then be lifted back into the car, above the level of his chest.

The treatment of shock at the roadside.

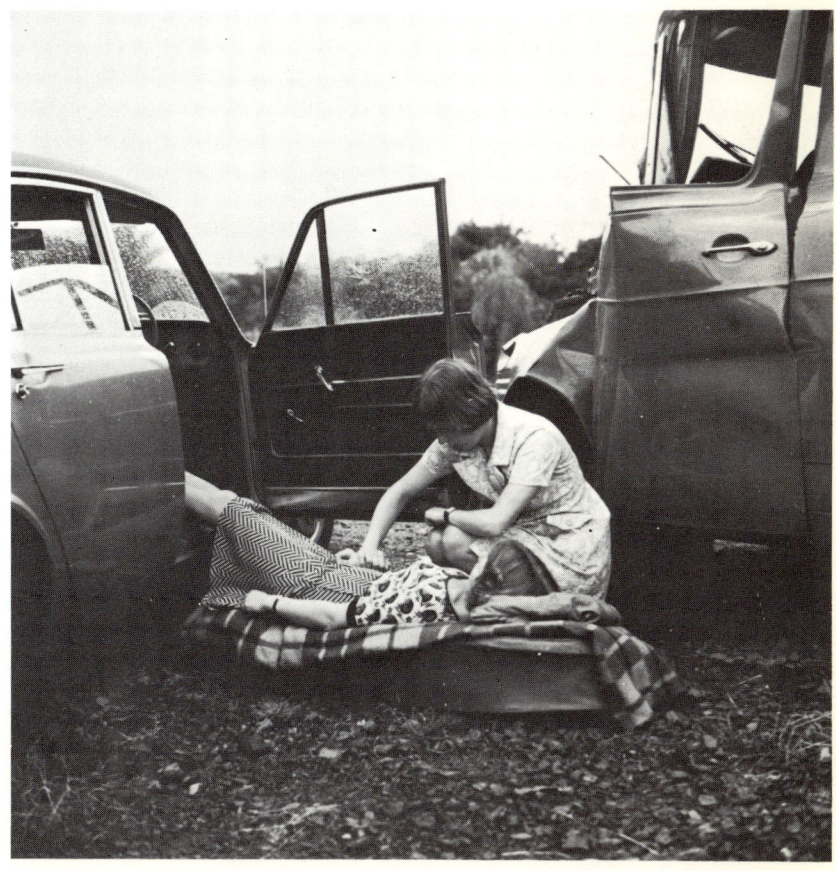

11
Poisoning

Cases of poisoning are not at all uncommon and can be very frightening. To be confronted suddenly by someone who has swallowed a substance which may cause death unless the correct treatment is immediately forthcoming, is a desperate situation, likely to terrify even a self-possessed first-aider. Fortunately, as we shall see, the emergency is often not quite so urgent as it seems. Begin by deciding whether the victim has taken some corrosive such as strong acid, or caustic soda. If he has, his lips and mouth will be burned and he is likely to be in severe pain. This is the first and really urgent rule: *when a poison is a corrosive, dilute it as quickly as possible by giving a lot of water*. Then the situation can be considered in rather more leisurely fashion. (Toxic fumes are discussed on page 57 and it is assumed that the reader is unlikely to have to deal with criminal poisoning.) The cases you will encounter will fall into two categories:

a   when the substance has been taken deliberately that is, because the patient was in a depressed or confused state. In such circumstances, it will usually be a medicine which has been correctly prescribed, in small doses, to relieve pain or anxiety or as a sedative. It is now fairly uncommon for would-be suicides to take other, more unpleasant and less easily swallowed substances but, occasionally of course, almost anything may be taken.

b   when the swallowing has been accidental, any of a very wide variety of poisons may be involved. Children eat tablets which they mistake for sweets and people of all ages may drink from bottles which do not contain the beverages which their colour, shape or label suggest.

AN OVERDOSE OF MEDICINE

The first situation, in which the poison is an overdose of some medicine, is seen more frequently. Certain features usually enable the first-aider to recognise it easily – the patient is often known to be affected by some nervous disorder, and may tell you what drug he has swallowed. Even when he is found alone and unconscious, there may be a note or an empty medicine container nearby. Bottles which have contained spirits are also significant, not only because a would-be suicide often drinks them with whatever tablets he swallows, but also because alcohol intensifies the action of some drugs. A glass of whisky, on top of an otherwise medicinal quantity of some sedatives may convert it into an overdose.

The patient may be seen within a few minutes, in which case he will still be conscious. A stage of excitement, sometimes almost of mania, can follow. Then there is an increasing drowsiness, and a lapse into unconsciousness. The rate at which these changes occur, and the depth of the subsequent coma, will depend on the quantity and type of the sedative taken. Few substances, however, cause fatal collapse in less than an hour; even large doses of the sedatives commonly prescribed frequently do not prove fatal the same day – an important and reassuring thought for the first-aider.

TREATMENT

If the patient is conscious, try to make him sick. Removing the tablets from his body before they are absorbed will prevent their harmful effects – and even if only part of the overdose is vomited, the risk of serious consequences is reduced. Vomiting, unfor-

tunately, is not always easy to induce. The simplest method –
thrusting one or two fingers down the patient's throat – works
well with a child but is less effective with a confused adult who is
bigger than the first-aider. It may be necessary to enlist help to
hold down the patient, and then to use one hand to thrust a
folded handkerchief, or the corner of a book into his mouth to
avoid being bitten. This improvised gag is wedged between his
back teeth in one angle of the mouth, while the fingers of the
other hand are pushed well down the throat.

When this has been done, or if it is unsuccessful, give a strong
solution of ordinary salt. A couple of tablespoons to a cup of
(preferably) warm water is the ideal strength but do not waste
time measuring out exact quantities, or trying to remember what
they should be. Just stir a very generous quantity of salt – too
much will do no harm, but too weak a solution will not produce
the desired result. Once the patient has vomited, let him have two
or three cupfuls of ordinary tap-water, and then make him sick
again. He may not appreciate your efforts, but you are washing
out any solid material – tablets, capsules etc. – which still remain
in his stomach. Remember two important rules which apply to
every case of poisoning, whatever the substance involved :
1   Always consult a doctor when anything has been swallowed
    which was not intended for consumption, or has been
    swallowed in larger quantities than were intended. Many
    substances in everyday use have no immediate effect when
    taken, but can prove fatal after several hours, or even days, of
    apparent well-being.
2   Keep carefully any vomited material. Collect it in a basin or a
    bucket. Do not allow the patient to be sick over a toilet, and
    preserve everything which he throws up. Its analysis may
    give invaluable assistance when deciding exactly what has
    been taken, and in what quantities.
If the patient is not conscious, or very drowsy, forget about making
him sick. (Any attempt to induce vomiting is likely to be followed
by inhalation of either the salt solution or the stomach contents,

into the air passages, and could cause death by choking.) Forget, too, about giving hot coffee or other stimulants, such as whisky, for the same reason. Efforts to rouse the patient or to keep him awake by dragging him up and down the room do no good, and may overtax a failing circulation.

Instead, place him in the position, previously described and illustrated on page 46, for an unconscious casualty and ensure that he can breathe easily. If his breathing becomes very shallow, or intermittent, be prepared to give mouth-to-mouth respiration, and to continue with this until medical help arrives.

ACCIDENTAL SWALLOWING

When we come to accidental poisoning, few general rules hold good. This is because almost any substance, liquid or solid, may be swallowed by a child and, though an adult is much less liable to accidental poisoning, he may very well drain, at a single gulp and by error, any fluid standing in a tumbler, a teacup, or a bottle which once held beer or lemonade. The liquids most commonly involved are domestic bleach, washing and cleaning solutions, and white spirit. Most of these fluids are so irritating, or taste so unpleasant, that the person immediately recognises his mistake. If more than one or two drops have been swallowed, however, the first-aider should try to make him sick, using one of the methods described on page 86 for an overdose of tablets. Then, after giving the patient a drink of milk or water, he should repeat the process (to wash out any traces of the poison which were not vomited on the first occasion).

Do not try to make the patient sick if his mouth and tongue have been burned. Their surface will turn brown or white, and look 'dead', suggesting that a corrosive substance, such as hydrochloric acid or caustic soda, has been swallowed. The act of vomiting may burst the stomach walls, leading to a very dangerous leakage of its contents into the abdomen at large. It is often said that vomiting should not be induced in corrosive poisoning 'because the poison burns the gullet a second time as it comes up'. This is irrelevant and untrue. The surface of the gullet is tanned by the first exposure to the poison and, even if severely damaged by that, would suffer only slight harm from the second one. Even if this were not so, the advantages of getting any corrosive out of the body as quickly as possible are so obvious that vomiting would be a good idea if it were not for this grave risk of perforation.

Remember that corrosive poisoning is one of the most urgent emergencies in the whole of first aid. Give something to dilute the poison immediately – water, milk, even urine, or the contents of the nearest pond or puddle. Keep giving the patient some such fluid and summon professional assistance as quickly as possible. Meanwhile, treat the profound shock which often develops (see pages 42–3), until this help arrives.

12
Emergency midwifery

Only a small percentage of babies are brought into this world by doctors and midwives. The first-aider who is called to a woman in labour should remember that, though it may be a novel experience for him, he is not exactly making history! If he is still apprehensive, and his patient is having her first child, he should keep in mind that her labour is likely to be long rather than short, so a doctor or midwife may well arrive before the baby does. This consolation may be denied him if his patient has had several babies before but he then has an advantage in that the mother, at least, has some experience.

A woman does not always know when labour has begun and 'false alarms' are common. Someone who is having abdominal pains at frequent, regular intervals and has a bloodstained watery discharge, probably is about to give birth. Initially the pains are ten or fifteen minutes apart but gradually become continuous. During this first stage, encourage the patient to rest and, between her pains, to relax as much as possible. Meanwhile, collect towels, soap and warm water. Find three pieces of tape (or bandage) each nine or ten inches long, and a pair of scissors. Cover a couch or a mattress with a raincoat or newspaper, then wash and scrub your hands.

When the pains increase in frequency and intensity, the patient gets an urge to contract her muscles and push. She should now lie on her back and bend up her legs. It may help if she braces these against for example, the foot of the bed. As each pain occurs, encourage her to take a deep breath, and hold it. The baby's head will now begin to stretch the skin round the entrance to the vagina. The first-aider should press on the head during the pains just hard enough to prevent the skin splitting or the baby being harmed by a violent expulsion. Grasp the baby's head and shoulders as these appear, and ease them out gently. The baby will be moist and very slippery. Raise it by the legs and clear any mucus from its mouth with a swab of cotton-wool or any clean cloth.

The baby will be joined to its mother by the umbilical cord, running from its navel to the afterbirth (placenta) which, at this stage, is still inside the womb. You need take no further action for about ten or fifteen minutes, during which time the afterbirth may be spontaneously expelled. At the end of this period, whether or not it has appeared, tie two pieces of tape very firmly round the umbilical cord (which has a fleshy, rather gelatinous, consistency and is about as thick as a man's finger). One piece should be about six inches from the navel, the other about twelve. Use a pair of scissors to cut the cord between these two ligatures. (During the first few days of life, the stump of cord running to the baby's navel shrivels and falls off). Then 'back up' the ligature, on the length of cord joined to the baby, by fastening another round the cord, but a little closer to the navel. This done, the baby should be wrapped in a towel, or some other dry cloth and placed in a suitable cot or box in a comfortable warm room. (Chilling of the baby is always a risk of confinement in awkward places, but take care not to asphyxiate it or allow it to get too warm).

If the mother continues to bleed at all heavily, before or after the placenta comes away, massage her abdomen gently and raise the foot of the bed. Keep the placenta, and any towels which indicate how much bleeding has accompanied the delivery, for the doctor or midwife to see.

Your first aid kit

The contents of this must depend on where it is likely to be used. Most householders can lay their hands on some clean handkerchiefs, a few strips of linen and a pair of scissors, and need store those together only as a matter of convenience. A group of people setting off into a very desolate country, for days or weeks on end, would be ill-advised to proceed without a comprehensive set of dressings and simple medicines. Any motorist may find himself faced with an emergency which he must treat with only the equipment in his own car. This should include at least the following items, preferably stored in a case or haversack which can be taken out and carried some distance, not kept loose in a glove compartment or door pocket.

  6 triangular bandages

  6 assorted roller bandages (from 6 in. to 2 in. wide. Crepe bandages are easier to use than cotton ones, but not so cheap —even so, have at least two, 6 in. and 3 in., of these)

  2 packets of gauze and/or of lint

  2 packets of cotton-wool

  1 1-inch roll of adhesive strapping

selection of small prepared adhesive dressings ('Band aid' or similar)

pair of scissors (Ideally, two pairs: one very large, for cutting clothing, and a small pair for dressings)

pair of tweezers (These should have very fine points, which meet accurately; they are rather expensive.)

12 safety-pins (in sizes ranging from the largest to the smallest easily obtainable)

torch

bottle of Paracetamol ('Panadol') tablets

small bottle of liquid paraffin or castor-oil

small bowl, and some soap or surgical detergent (in case you
need to cleanse a wound, and can find some suitable water)

If it is to be kept in a car this outfit need not be very compact.
If, however, you intend to carry some or all of these items when
hiking, for instance, it is worth shopping round for bandages,
wool and gauze compressed into very small packages. Government surplus dealers sometimes sell 'First Field Dressings', or
'Shell Dressings', which are an ideal basis for any emergency kit.

Learning more : suggestions for further reading

Of the many books on first aid, one 'First Aid. The Authorised Manual of St John Ambulance, St Andrew's Ambulance Association, and the British Red Cross Society' must be read by all serious students of the subject because it is so comprehensive and so widely accepted as the standard text.

Principles for 'First Aid for the Injured' by H. Proctor and P. S. London (Butterworths) covers the same ground but is concerned with the physiological and anatomical results of injury, and the reasons underlying established doctrines. It demands some previous knowledge on the part of the reader but is ideal for the student who, having learned what to do, now wants to know why it is done.

Another book 'The Ship Captain's Medical Guide' (HMSO) is unique, in that it affords instruction about what to do when the customary advice 'and send for a doctor' is useless. Though designed for seafarers, most of its contents are equally applicable to any group of people, large or small, who will be living in isolation.

If you are learning first aid for use in such situations, you should certainly attend one of the short lecture courses held regularly, all over the country, by the organisations mentioned above. The opportunity of discussing points about which you may be doubtful, of seeing the various techniques demonstrated by an expert, and of proving your own proficiency by taking an examination for a very widely recognised certificate, will increase your competence and confidence.

Anyone interested in first aid should remember, however, that it is a subject where experience is more important than theoretical study. Such experience is best acquired by joining one of the societies. Then, after appropriate instruction, he will be assigned to duties at public functions where there will almost always be some demand on his services.

Index